JOURNAL
OF A
CAREGIVER

*Caregiver to an
Alzheimer's Patient*

Charles H. Morris

Charles H. Morris

JOURNAL OF A CAREGIVER

Charles H. Morris

This book has been written to assist others who have a family member or friend with one of the forms of Alzheimer's disease. If it is helpful to those to cope with this devastating disease, I will feel God has allowed me to walk this way for a purpose. The contents may be used in any way to help or comfort those who are caregivers.

If any of the material is used, acknowledgement of the source will be appreciated.

Additional copies are available for the cost of printing plus mailing by contacting the author at:

1900 Lauderdale Drive, Apt. A-319,
Richmond, Virginia 23233
Telephone 804-754-0341 or email c7em@erols.com

Printed in the United States of America by
BRENTWOOD CHRISTIAN PRESS
4000 BEALLWOOD AVENUE
COLUMBUS, GEORGIA 31904

DEDICATION

****

To my darling wife, ERICA. who through out life's experiences has displayed a deep and abiding faith in her Lord.

Today her only means of sharing that faith is her elegant grace and peace inspiring all who knew her in the past and challenging new friends to follow her example of the all-sufficient grace of her Lord in the midst of the worst of the worst diseases—Alzheimer's.

JOURNAL ENTRIES

APPRECIATION

I am humbled and grateful for the hundreds of responses I have received from the United States of America, Singapore, Malaysia, Indonesia, England, Philippine Islands and Australia about these entries. Your constant encouragement spurred me on to continue to expose my feelings and to proceed with publishing these entries in a book. Your prayer support anointed my ability to write and give birth to the book.

I thank my Lord that He has used these emotional outpourings to assist pastors and friends to assist others walking this same path. The pain is not removed but knowing that these entries have helped others makes the agony less severe.

I acknowledge with gratitude the financial contributions from my family, Dr. Eric E. Morris and Ambassador Greta Morris. My dear friend Miss Audrey Salzer, friend from missionary days, helped with the publishing cost. Our pioneering partners and Chinese brother and sister, Mr. and Mrs. Tsui See Chong, Sandakan, Sabah, Malaysia, contributed to the expense of mailing.

I am indebted to my Chinese son in the ministry, Dr. Isaac Yim Yee Sart, Petaling Jaya, Malaysia for arranged and financing the Asian edition of the book.

A big "thank you" to my spiritual brother, Russell Morris, who spent hours correcting grammar, syntax and spelling and making suggestions about how to make the book more readable.

I am deeply indebted to the professional health care persons at the Lakewood Manor Retirement Community who provided loving care for Erica releasing me to prepare the entries for publication.

I am indebted to my friend, David Jordan, whose expertise with the computer guided me in bringing the book to fruition.

I am grateful and gladly acknowledge the many poets, known and unknown, whose writings inspired and strengthened me in the journey of a caregiver.

I am indebted to David Seay, Editor-in-Chief of the *Mature Living* magazine, for encouraging me to write the March 2004 article for the magazine and to publish the book.

I appreciate Lisa P. Gwyther of the Duke Medical Center, for granting me permission to quote from her book You Are One of Us.

I am indebted to Zondervan Publishing House for permission to quote from the New International Version of the Bible.

INTRODUCTION

THE DESTROYER

Alzheimer's disease is the master destroyer. It destroys the afflicted. More than four millions persons in the U.S.A. have the disease. It is the fourth leading cause of death, after heart disease, cancer and stroke. It can afflict persons as young as 40 years of age. It is not necessarily a part of the aging process but this devastating disease disables 10% of all people over 65 and nearly 50% of people over 85. It is a progressively debilitating, degenerative disorder of the brain. It results in gradual loss of cognition, including memory, language and comprehension. It cause decline in the ability to function normally in such things as decision-making, judgment, attention, speaking and personality.

Dr. Alois Alzheimer, a German physician, first described the disease in 1906. The brain of the afflicted person will show "neurofibrillary tangles" (twisted fragments of protein within nerve cells that clog up the cell), "neuritic plaques" (abnormal clusters of dead and dying nerve cells, other brain cells, and protein), and "senile plaques" (areas where products of dying nerve cells have accumulated around protein). The brain cells die and are not replaced. Alzheimer's disease is a complicated illness and each individual case is unique. There are treatments for the disease but no cure has yet been discovered. A medical doctor is the best source of information on treatment.

The cause of the disease is not known. People with family history of the disease are considered at risk. Brain tumors, head injuries and nutritional deficiencies may also be contributing causes. It is not preventable. It is not reversible. It is not contagious. It is not known to be painful. It is not to be ashamed. The patient need not be hidden away. The symptoms are delineated but are not chronological; Each patient may react differently to what is happening to him/her. Not every person experiences every symptom at the same time or place in the categories. Some symptoms overlap or vary when they occur.

The disease is usually described in three stages—

MILD: Between two and four years.

MODERATE: Between one to ten years.

SEVERE: Between one to three years.

NOTE: Alzheimer's Association is the most reliable source of information and assistance.

Alzheimer's destroys the family. It is the most devastating disease known. When it casts its blanket over the patient it disrupts, disturbs and destroys normal family routine and relational well-being. It exacts its toll on the physical, emotional, financial and relations of the family. When Erica was diagnosed with the disease I was devastated. I have been a pastor and missionary for over 61 years. I now am a caregiver to my best friend and beloved wife. Alzheimer's has handcuffed her intellect, competency, comprehension, creativity and talents. I am deprived of stimulating conversation, shared prayer times and thought provoking insights, The pain of watching her being taken from me bit by bit is heartbreaking and depressing. I determined for my own sanity and peace of mind to -

√ Learn everything I could about the disease.

√ Be honest, open and forthright with family, friends and myself.

√ Provide the best care possible for Erica.

√ Seek daily guidance and strength to cope from God's Word and prayer.

√ Write a journal about what is happening to Erica and me.

√ Share and minister to others in the same situation.

THE BEGINNING

MARCH 3, 2000

The tires squealed burning black marks on the road. Metal ripped open the left front side of the car. Air bags popped. Glass shattered. Doors were twisted. Tires deflated. Sirens whined toward the accident to gather the injured and scream away to the hospital.

Erica had been shopping at her favorite mall. She was hurrying to pick me up at church. She sped through the red light. The truck plowed into our car. The telephone jangled in my office. An unknown woman uttered the chilling words, "Your wife has been in an accident. I think she is o.k. She wants you to come". A fellow staff member rushed me to the scene. Erica was dazed and confused. The police were quizzing her and writing a report. Erica remembered nothing. She had no obvious injuries. She refused to go to the hospital.

The next day I took her to the family doctor to be examined. The doctor suspected a neck injury. A cat scan confirmed that she had broken the second vertebra at the base of her skull. The neurosurgeon was amazed she was alive. He prescribed an Aspen collar to hold her head stiff. She wore it for 13 months. The collar limited her vision. She missed a step and fell breaking her pelvis on the right side. For 37 days her body responded to rest and therapy. Erica struggled to learn to walk again. She did fine. While making a hospital visit with me two women crowded her off the sidewalk. She fell and broke the left side of her pelvis. Since then the walker and wheelchair have been her companions.

On May 15, 2001 her family doctor began to note dementia. He recommended seeing a psychiatrist. On August 22, 2002 the psychiatrist gave her a battery of test. He blurted out the chilling words "She has Alzheimer's disease. She has had it for some time. I can't do anything for her." He felt that the disease blocked out her memory of where she was, causing the auto accident. The brain injury and trauma probably hurried the disease along.

I determined I would take care of her. I soon began to learn what that meant. To help me cope with Erica's condition and my own personal needs I began to write out my frustrations and emotions. Writing was my therapy. These writings are very personal. They are the heart cry of a distraught husband caring for a wife I love more than life itself.

As Erica's condition became known people began to pray for us. They began to inquire, "How are you coping?" "I am writing out my feelings and what God is saying to me." I replied. They asked, "Would you share your writing with me? I have a family member or friend who has Alzheimer's disease and I need help in knowing how to cope." They shared with friends, family and their pastors. The pastors wrote for copies as a mean of helping members in their congregations. I don't know where or to whom they have gone. I don't know who has been helped by my confessions of heart and frustration of spirit. This is not important.

I continue to learn all I can. The knowledge gained rips at my emotions. Pain, apprehension and hope rise and fall with the knowledge. Each day I find Erica in a different mood. My emotions daily are on a roller coaster. Some days I am exhilarated. Other days I hurt and am frustrated. I search to find ways to minister to Erica and others in the unit. I daily look for the fulfillment of the promise *"And we know that in all things God works for the good of those who love him, who have been called according to his purpose"*. (Romans 8:28) I pray for peace for myself and others who are helped by the journal to say with confidence *"What, then, shall we say in response to this? If God is for us, who can be against us"*(Romans 8:31).

BECOMING A BABY AGAIN

JANUARY 20, 2003

Alzheimer's disease turns back the clock of life. It reverses the stream of growing in the ability to function. It reverts the patient to being a child again. The longer one suffers with the disease the more the regression. My darling Erica is daily turning back into a baby.

She often needs to be spoon-fed. When she does want to try to feed herself she holds the fork or spoon like a baby trying to master the technique of eating. She needs encouragement to eat the correct food. She has to be prevented from putting the wrong things in her mouth. She must wear a bib because often she misses her mouth. At times, like a baby, she refuses to open her mouth. She will purse her lips or clamp her teeth so food cannot be put in her mouth. She will jerk her head back and refuse to eat. She will spit out what she doesn't want. She will hold the food in her mouth and refuse to swallow. As I watch her I see our sons at this same stage of life. This is so excruciatingly painful to me. I pray every moment for patience and understanding. This is not my sweet Erica. She is not responsible for her actions. She doesn't understand what she is doing. At times she grows impatient with me as I am trying to help her. She would never want to be like this. O, Lord, help me help her in her greatest hour of need.

Erica has no idea where she is going. She clings to my hand and trusts me to lead or direct her. My arm is her security. My felt love is her strength.

Erica, who was once brilliant and fluent in three languages, has shrunk from stimulating and ongoing conversation to sentences, to a few words, to nothing. Like a baby she points instead of trying to formulate words. Her beautiful handwriting is now just a scribble. Once an avid reader, now she cannot read. A complete picture of babyhood.

The disease makes the patient incontinent. She must be diapered, bathed and changed. She cannot perform the ordinary bathroom activities. She no longer can comb her hair, brush her teeth, choose or put on jewelry and apply her make up. She depends on me or the health care aide to choose her wardrobe and dress her. She is our darling baby. We are grateful we can perform these things for her as an act of love. The agony of seeing this beautiful person shrink into baby hood is very devastating. Knowing that she can't relearn these normal activities of life is like a sword piercing my soul.

Scientists and doctors are perplexed. Unlike a child eager to learn, grow and advance, she is going backward. Like a hurricane the wild disease rips apart her ability to regain what she once was. She is not responsible for who she is now. If she knew her condition she would be unhappy.

In desperation this morning I cried to the Lord, "Give me a word for today!" The Spirit directed my attention to Matthew 18, where the Lord Jesus was speaking about children. He said, *"They will enter the kingdom (v.5). They are greatest in the kingdom (v. 4). They always behold the face of the Father (v.10) and whoever welcomes a little child like these in my name welcomes me (v.5)".* To receive, care for and love these is to receive him. He warns *"See that you do not look down on one of these little ones" (v.10)* for *"your Father in heaven is not willing that any of these little ones should be lost. (v.14)*

Erica can't formulate words to pray audibly. I believe she is nearer to her Lord and feels His presence stronger now than ever. It is my privilege to be her shepherd and lead her. My dearest Erica is my baby girl. It is to be my joy to do for her the things that I did for our sons My daily prayer is for strength, grace and patience to be her caregiver. I rejoice I can still cuddle and cradle her in my arms I. I pray for strength as I struggle in the darkness of this evil disease. My prayer for Erica is voiced in the third verse of the ancient hymn *Away in a Manger*,

"Be near me. Lord Jesus, I ask you to stay
Close by me forever, and love me. I pray;
Bless all the dear children in Thy tender care.
And fit us for heaven and to live with Thee There"

John Thomas McFarland

TEARS

FEBRUARY 1, 2003

Alzheimer's disease disables the mind of the afflicted. The mental distress to the caregiver produces tears and weeping. Frequently tears from my eyes course down my cheek, not from physical pain but from emotional hurting. Each day I struggle to understand what is happening to Erica. I understand somewhat what the Psalmist felt, *"You have fed them with the bread of tears; you have made them drink tears by the bowlful"* (80:5). *"My tears have been my food day and night"* (42:3). Voltaire was correct when he said, "Tears are the silent language of grief". Words are throttled in my throat by tears when I attempt to talk to others about Erica's condition. Dreaming about her causes the fountains to burst forth and wet my pillow. I understand the tears of frustration. Jesus wept over what might have been (Matthew 23:37). He wept over the inevitable to come (Luke 19:41-44). Jesus wept over the loss of love of a loved one (John 11:35,36). Memories rush in unbidden and the tears flow. The depth of my love for Erica and her inability to return that love brings—*"great distress and anguish of heart and with many tears"* (2 Corinthians 2:4). My helplessness to change her condition or alleviate her losses or bring healing brings tears of frustration.

A restless night propelled me from my bed seeking help. I picked up the book *Tears in God's Bottle* by my friend, Dr. Wayne Ewing. I re-read how he wept over the death of his wife, Ann, who died with Alzheimer's disease, when she was only 60 years of age. He wrote of how lonely he was. I know the tears of loneliness. I know how I ache to her Erica's voice. I know the tears of an empty room. I know the tears of helplessness as I face the inevitable.

I felt led to turn to Philippians 1:19-25. I was inspired by the insights and courage as Paul faced the inevitable. Erica has

Alzheimer's disease. The symptoms have been identified. The progress has been documented. Timing of anticipated reaction is projected.

The thief, Alzheimer's, is stealing Erica from me bit by bit each day. I know we all will die, but when the symptoms are spelled out so graphically I weep as I see them coming to fruition. The sword of anguish twists in my soul as I struggle to understand her needs and try to minister to her. Selfishly, I ask "What about me?". I cannot imagine being separated after our wonderful 61 years together.

Paul's attitude spoke to my agonizing soul. He writes, *"Yes, I will continue to rejoice. For I know that through your prayers and the help given by the Spirit of Jesus Christ, what has happened to me will turn out for my deliverance"* (1:18, 19). As Paul faced the inevitable his prayer was *"I will in no way be ashamed, but will have sufficient courage so that now as always Christ will be exalted in my body* (v. 20).

While awaiting the inevitable Paul said there were two things he was to do. First, he was to go on living (v. 22). This shook me up. Erica and I had always said we wished we could die together in an accident. Now I realize that Alzheimer's disease may swing the scythe of death and separate us. One will be left alone. It could be me that is the one left. The frightening thought was "Then what?" Paul's words thundered in my heart, "For to me, to live is Christ. If I am to go on living in the body, this will mean fruitful labor for me" (vs. 22,23).

Secondly, is the question "Why? and for what purpose?" Paul says that he and I are to go on ministering. He longed to be with Christ *"It is more necessary for you that I remain in the body. Convinced of this, I know that I will remain, and I will continue with all of you for your progress and joy in the faith, so that through my being with you again your joy in Christ Jesus will overflow on account of me"* (vs. 24-26).

15

Paul's words dried my tears. He encouraged me to face the inevitable with anticipation that my journey through the thicket of this disease could be helpful to others. God did not cause the situation. So the situation must be used to assist others. My daily prayer is for grace, strength and faith to believe that in the Lord's graciousness there is a ministry yet ahead.

I am encouraged that in God's tenderness He will *"Record my lament; list my tears on your scroll (put my tears in your bottle)— Are they not in your record?* (Psalm 56:8). I was assured with His promise *"By this I know that God is for me. In God, whose word I praise in the Lord, whose word I praise—in God I trust; I will not be afraid. What can man do to me?"* Psalm 56:9-11). Alzheimer's will not have the final answer. We are assured the time is coming when the Lamb *"will lead them to springs of living water. And God will wipe away every tear from their eyes. There will be no more death or mourning or crying or pain. For the old order of things has passed away"* (Revelation 7:17,21:4).

SILENCE

FEBRUARY 5, 2003

Ecclesiastes 3:7 says, *"There is a time for everything. A time to be silent and a time to speak"*. At times we crave a little silence. When the silence is imposed it s not golden! It can be devastating! As the hideous, debilitating plaque becomes thicker on the nerves controlling cognition, memory, knowledge and movements the silence becomes louder. It is more obvious and oppressive with each day. There are days when silence reeks to where I can almost touch it and smell its presence.

For over 60 years our times of praying together for family, friends, co-workers, the ill and troubled and ourselves were a daily joy. Recalling her words, I remember that *"Pleasant words are a honeycomb, sweet to the soul and healing to the bones"* (Proverbs 16:24). Now, when I ask Erica to pray, she either mumbles, "you pray" or begins and then stops. The words cannot come. I weep with anguish over my beloved whose prayer life has been a teacher of righteousness to me. Her words to me were *"A word aptly spoken is like apples of gold in settings of silver"* (Proverbs 25:11). At times, when I become aware that Erica is troubled and I inquire, I am met with a vacant stare, a shake of the head or "I can't tell you". This pierces my soul like a sword and I am frustrated and wounded because I cannot respond to her need. Now when I desperately need her good advice there is only the silence of "do what you think is best". I don't know what is best, and I need her so badly.

The Greek word for "muzzle" means "putting to silence or subduing to silence," Her beautiful alto voice has sung in choirs and groups in more than one language in many parts of the world. Her speaking voice has inspired and encouraged crowds of people. Now her voice is seldom heard. She has been my confidant, sharing my concerns, giving helpful advice, correcting my mistakes and commending my achievements. Now—only silence. My whole being aches to hear her voice.

I turned today to Revelation 5:9-14 and rejoiced at the time when spontaneously she and others will sing before the throne of the Lord. Please Lord do not let it come too soon! I need her so badly.

I regret the times when I did not converse enough with her. I pray for all to value the sound of a loved one's voice while it is still possible to hear it. I pray that none of us will be silent to those we love while they are still able to comprehend and respond. I pray for myself to have patience to continue to share with Erica, tell her of my love for her, and eagerly look for the responses she may give.

LAUGHTER

FEBRUARY 7, 2003

As I struggle through the brambles of the devastating Alzheimer's disease, which has abducted Erica mind from the realm of the past and made the future a fog of uncertainty, there seems little to laugh about. The cloud of fear and apprehension make it difficult to crack the hardness of spirit and gloom of the face. I thank the Lord this morning we experienced laughter.

Yesterday was a good day! We traveled 30 miles to visit a dying friend in a part of Virginia we had never seen before. Erica thoroughly enjoyed being out and seeing the countryside. In the somber hospital room, with the tubes and gasping of my friend, the wife, daughter and friends recalled times of sweet relationships between us and them. Spontaneously we laughed. Erica laughed. The tension snapped and all were at peace.

On the way home we stopped for Chinese food. She was happy! The perplexing frown on her forehead relaxed. Later as I was helping her prepare for bed something about brushing her teeth struck the cord of hilarity. She laughed. I joined with her and we hugged and laughed together.

As I reflected over the day I was reminded of the words of Bildad to Job in the midst of his testing time. *"He will yet fill your mouth with laughter and your lips with shouts of joy (Job 8:21).* There is a time to weep and a time to laugh (Ecclesiastes 3:4).

The Hebrew word means "an outburst of gladness--a pleasurable surprise".

Curiously I thought "how can we laugh with this hideous disease grinding away at us?" Then I remember the words of Jesus *"Blessed are you who weep now: for you will laugh" (Luke 6:21).*

19

Today Psalm 126:2 has a new meaning for me. Israel returning from the darkness of captivity could say *"Our mouths were filled with laughter, our tongues with songs of joy. The Lord has done great things for us and we are filled with joy"*. Like a shaft of sunshine I saw that God had given us the hammer of laughter to break the chain of gloom and doom that was surrounding Erica and me. There must be time to laugh at ourselves and let the disease know that though it crushes the mental capacities it will not crush the spirit of joy in each of us. Our Lord has reminded us *"Do not be afraid of those who kill the body, but cannot kill the soul." (Matthew 10:28).*

I pray for myself that whereas I weep alone for her and myself I will not fail to laugh and be full of joy because of my Lord and supporting friends. I am determined to be intent on looking for things of joy as Erica struggles, I want to laugh with her. I want to cause her to laugh. I want to bring pure joy to her. I want to see her laugh. I want to make her yesterdays "a dream of happiness and every tomorrow a vision of hope". I want to help make her life of the NOW one of laughter and joy.

CONFUSION

FEBRUARY 12, 2003

Alzheimer's disease brings confusion. Erica is confused about what day it is, what time it is, where she is, where she is going and for what purpose. The doctors are confused about how the disease reacts in various people and thus have no hopeful remedies. I am confused about what to do next, how to minister to her and others. I am confused about decisions I must make with each dawning day. There is an endless circle of confusion. There are many ways to respond and react to confusion.

Often I am surprised at myself. While assisting Erica and struggling to encourage her to do the things she needs and must do, a song will bubble up and I will begin to sing or whistle. "Just a minute", I think. "This is a time of confusion full of unsolvable problems. This insidious disease is ripping Erica away from me physically, mentally and emotionally. Is this a time to sing? Or is this a song birthed out of pain?"

This morning I felt led to read Exodus 32-34. Moses is on Mt. Sinai. This is a story of confusion. The people were confused. Moses had been gone too long. The confused people said, *"This fellow Moses who brought us up out of Egypt, we don't know what has happened to him"*. (Exodus 32:23) They reacted by turning away from God and began singing and indulging in revelry as they created and worshipped a hand made idol and running about wildly.

Moses is coming down the mountain from an exciting time with God. Clutched in both hands were the two tablets. *"To the work of God; the writing was the writing of God, engraved on the Tablets" (Exodus 32:16)*. He danced down the mountain with the ten rules by which mankind could live a life well pleasing to God. He was jolted to hear the sound of singing. He said to Joshua, *"It*

21

is not the sound of victory, it is not the sound of defeat; it is the sound of singing that hear"(Exodus 32:18).

Moses was confused, *"He threw the tablets out of his hands, breaking them in pieces at the foot of the mountain"* (Exodus 32:19). He reacted in anger. He felt betrayed by the Lord and the people. After all he had been through leading the people out of bondage--now this! After all he had done for the people in the name of the Lord--now this!

In anger he smashed the writing of God. He ground the idol to powder and made the people drink the waters of bitterness made from the powder (Exodus 32:20). The unbelief and confusion among the people triggered singing and dancing. Not the right time! Not the right place! Not the right song! This is one reaction to confusion. Is there not a better reaction to confusion?

God is still at work. Moses cooled down and prayed, *"Teach me your ways so I may know you and continue to find favor with you"* (Exodus 33:13). The Lord replied *"My Presence will go with you, and I will give you rest. I will cause my goodness to pass in front of you, and I will proclaim my name, the Lord, in your presence"* (Exodus 33:14,19). God promised to give a new set of the writings. (Exodus 34:1). The requirement was for Moses to *"Present yourself to me"* (Exodus 34:1,2). This promise gives birth to a better reaction to confusion. It causes a song of praise to roll up out of the soul. Out of the Exodus experience David wrote, *"The Lord's unfailing love surrounds the man who trusts in Him. Rejoice in the Lord and be glad, you righteous; sing, all you who are upright in heart"(Psalm 32:10,11).*

This cauterizing disease cannot obliterate the song of my righteous Erica. Tucked in her memory are the songs of faith. Spontaneously to the radio or in church the words come tumbling out. The written words she may not comprehend, but this confusing disease cannot obliterate the words engraved on the tablets of her heart.

22

Is it right for this dreaded disease to do this to my beloved who has served God faithfully since a teen as a pastor's wife, missionary, counselor, teacher and soul winner? NO! But that changes nothing! It is here! How do I react? Lord, help me to continue to sing. Help the overflow of her heart continue to feel the songs of faith.

Then there will be victory over confusion. Help me in my helplessness and confusion to be confident that *"God is not a God of disorder but of peace"* (I Corinthians 14:33). Help me to sing with the Psalmist, *"I am still confident of this: I will see the goodness of the Lord in the land of the living. Wait for the Lord; be strong and take heart and wait for the Lord—all you who hope in the Lord"* (Psalm 27:13,14; 31:24).

MY VALENTINE

FEBRUARY 16, 2003

This has been Valentine Week--the Week of LOVE. It has not been a good week. Different events clutching at the ragged edges of Erica's mind, inability to communicate or comprehend and the struggle of movement from one place to another have taken their toll.

In 1999 Carol Lynn Pearson wrote a small book **WHAT LOVE IS**. The subtitle is *A Fable for Our Times*. She intends it to *"present this life long story--one that transcends the bonds of illness, age, unemployment and more"*. **Love is not a <u>fable!</u> IT** IS THE LIFE BREATH OF EXISTENCE. Each person who loves will be tested. I Corinthians 13 is the test. How am I measuring up in this time of wrestling with the ripping disease of Alzheimer's?

Driving back home after one of the week's events I asked, "Are you happy?" Erica replied, "When I am with you I am happy!" She seems to know that all is not well but clings to the NOW and in that NOW there is a sense of security. This security is bound up in the KNOWN. The KNOWN is usually centered in a person. With Erica I am that person. She is in love with me. The love has grown in depth over 62 years. The love has been welded together by good and the not so good. She once told me that she fell in love with me when I was willing to walk in the rain with her along stormy Lake Michigan in Chicago when we were in school. That drippy experience increased to a downpour of happiness, love, dependability and security. Through the years the flame of love grew hotter as we endured the ravages of life. Song of Solomon 8:6,7 says, *"Love is as strong as death, its jealousy unyielding as the grave. It burns like a blazing fire, like a mighty flame. Many waters cannot quench love; rivers cannot wash it away. If one were to give all the wealth of his house for love, it would be utterly scorned"*. As I care for Erica I find a new depth of love. As Tom Wilson says in his Ziggy cartoon, *"Love is a present that should never be left unopened"*. As the spin

24

of this dreaded disease whirls, the present is opened in different ways. There is no pattern to follow--no pre-arranged response. To Erica it is my presence. It is her trust in my being there for her. It is the touch of the hand in her foggy search for reality. At night when we go to bed her hand gropes for my hand. She tightly clutches it until sleep relaxes her. If I try to move my hand too soon she tightens her grip. Sometimes when she awakens during the night I feel her searching for my hand. Only when she is able to feel my presence does she sleep. The last words I say to her are, "I love you". Her final words are, "I love you also".

I rejoice in the knowledge that there is a hand, much, much stronger than mine who says *"I give them eternal life, and they shall never perish; no one is able to snatch them out of my hand. My Father, who has given them to me, is greater than all; no one can snatch them out of my Father's hand. I and the Father are one"* John 10:28,29.

Love has built a bridge of security over the troubled waters of this dreadful disease. The oil of security and love poured into the disturbed mind of Erica bring serenity and peace. It is my privilege and joy to open the present of love and shower it upon her by acts of kindness, by my presence and by making her feel secure. When I am out of her sight she becomes agitated. When she doesn't see me she searches for me. Uneasiness drives her to find her security. I daily pray, "O Lord, give me the strength to be strong for one so weak. May my flame of love encircle her and bring her an experience of peace. I pray, as the floodwaters of Alzheimer's disease grow deeper, I will stand firm on the Rock, Christ Jesus, and hold her above the waters that are consuming her. Let me hold her hand as we climb the ragged mountain of this disease until she relaxes and touches a hand that will let her climb above the disease.

The writing is becoming blurred. The tears are breaking over the dam of my eyelids as I write. The hatred for this disease that is chipping away at my beloved Erica must be superceded by my love for her. My greatest earthly treasure is Erica, my valentine.

PATIENCE

FEBRUARY 26, 2003

I am not a patient person. Never have been. In the pastorate or on the mission field I wanted to hurry and finish one project so I could move on to another one. I want things to happen NOW and on time. I want things to take place as planned. I grow agitated waiting in lines at the post office, grocery store, gasoline pump and cafeteria. I fume inside at meetings where the participants get off the agenda and go chasing rabbits about irrelevant things. I dislike waiting in a doctor's office when the doctor doesn't keep the appointment time. I fret when airplanes don't keep their schedule. When I had cancer and two heart operations I fretted to get on with the treatment so I could get back to doing the things I felt needed to be done. At times I was so weak I could not stand and I should have learned patience, but it didn't take. I had yet to learn *"Patience is better than pride. Do not be quickly provoked in your spirit, for anger resides in the lap of fools" (Ecclesiastes 7:8,9).*

In August, 2002 Erica was diagnosed as having "severe dementia". The psychiatrist ran a variety of tests to access memory and thinking skills. She could respond to only 13 of 39. Physical examinations revealed no physical problems. The doctor said, "She has Alzheimer's disease. There is no cure. Medication may slow down the progress. She is among the more than 50% of the population over 80 years who has Alzheimer's disease". This shocking statement sent my mind reeling. It was almost more than I could take in. I thought, "How can this happen to some one as intelligent, alert and creative as Erica?" Impatiently I questioned the doctor for some encouraging, positive statement. There was none. Then I began to see why Paul's list of necessities to live through the rocky road of being a follower of Christ included--"love must be sincere... be devoted to one another... keep your spiritual fervor...be joyful in hope, **patient in affliction**, faithful in prayer" (Romans 12:9-13).

The word "**patience**" in the Greek means, "abiding under". Proverbs 14:29 *"A patient man has great understanding"*. I was faced with the task of understanding what it means to "abide under" that which I could not control, could not see a light at the end of the tunnel or organize a way out. I needed to "abide under" what is happening to my beloved. I must learn to be patient. My daily prayer now is "Lord, help me be patient". Scripture defines "patience": as being "long spirited". In almost all cases it refers to having this attitude while abiding under difficulty. Alzheimer's disease is the most difficult thing I have ever endured. Patience is needed when she doesn't want to eat or doesn't like what is there and she just looks in bewilderment at my efforts to feed her or just sits with her hands in her lap. Somehow the nerve cells have become disconnected and the message doesn't reach the part of the brain that moves the arms. The message doesn't get through. I am learning to wait patiently and then try again.

Before the disease she always encouraged me on our daily walks to go faster because it did more good. The walks have ended. She barely can shuffle one foot in front of the other. I pray for patience to walk more slowly. I pray for patience when I try to communicate with her and the abnormal cluster of dead and dying cells clogs up the skill to formulate words. I am devastated for I so want to hear her dialogue with me. I pray for patience to try to interpret what she cannot say. When I need her to perform the necessary bathroom activities and her limbs do not move or she reacts as a child might I pray for patience and wait. When she mumbles, "I don't want to". I pray for patience. I pray for patience as I offer her a choice of clothing to wear and she looks at me and says, "Whatever you want". James 1:2-4 says that trials are a test of faith to develop patience and patience *"must finish its work so that you may be mature and complete, not lacking anything"*. I squirm when James says," *Consider it pure joy... whenever- you face trials of many kinds"*. Patience indeed must finish its work for there to be seen any joy in Alzheimer's disease.

Paul in I Corinthians 13, lists 15 characteristics of love. The first (and perhaps the most important) is, **"love is patient."** Therein lies the triumphant fortitude that brings joy. Not the absence of murmuring but with a song of praise for what love can do. The next characteristic, **"love is kind"** or "sweet to all", moves me to be patient with my sweetheart as she has always been to all others and me.

I am despondent and pray, "O Lord, I am too weak for this. It is against all I am. Help me understand what Jesus meant when He said, *'In patience possess your soul'* (Luke 21:19 KJV)".

As Erica wanders down the unknown paths of Alzheimer's disease with me at her side I must learn to live the words of Psalm 37 where the psalmist calls for us to "fret not" (be not impatient). God reminds me that patience can be developed as I actively trust in the Lord; delight in the Lord; commit myself to the Lord and as I am still and wait patiently for Him.

"Lord, this is hard. Teach me how to look to you as my stronghold in trouble and my place of refuge. I fail daily, Lord, to be patient. Strengthen my faith so I will not fail Erica--will not offend whatever feelings are still operating. Help my love be as strong as life so that we can walk this path,

PRAYER

FEBRUARY 22, 2003

This is one of those hard weeks doctors said would come more and more frequently as the twisted fragments of protein clog up the nerve cells and neurotic abnormal clusters of dead and dying cells short circuit the brain. Erica is weak and trembling. She cannot stand without help. She fell this week and hurt herself but she is not able to form words to tell me where she hurts. She does not always comprehend what I am saying. Her motor skills are short-circuited. She needs help to do most everything. I am walking on the knife-edge of bewilderment. Her eyes and body movements tell me she is in trouble. I cannot seem to help her. My eyes are swimming. I can only cuddle her and tell her how much I love her. She replies "I love you too" as she drifts off into the pit of unresponsiveness. I am in despair. My eyes are swimming as I stand by helplessly. I pray *"Hear my prayer, O Lord, listen to my cry for help; be not deaf to my weeping"* (Psalm 39:12). I ask the Lord to unclouded my eyes so I can see clearly how to help. My heart is breaking. Where can I turn for help? I pray, *"Come, O Sovereign Lord and wipe away my tears"* (Isaiah 25:8), so I can be the caregiver I want to be. Where can I find help?

While drinking the dregs of despair Job 16:20 leaps out at me. *"My intercessor is my friend as my eyes pour our tears to God; on behalf of a man he pleads with God as a man pleads for his friend"*.

Thumbing through the responses to my requests for prayer I find email from ten states and several foreign countries. They cover all the time zones in America and virtually every time zone in the world. I am humbled that my friend, the Lord Jesus, *"always lives to intercede for me (Hebrews 7:25)* but I am profoundly moved that someone is praying for us every hour of the day and night. I feel your arms encircling us. I am deluged with a peace beyond understanding. I feel the prayers bouncing off heaven and falling

29

like raindrops into my spirit. Knowing that my intercessors are praying is like a soft handkerchief wiping away my tears.

Being prayed for is like nectar in a beautiful flower. In a week like this I touch the flower and am showered with the sweet nectar. I feel warm in the non-ending intensity of blessing from your prayers. I hear God interpreting into my searching soul prayers in Indonesian, Malaysian, Chinese, Indian, Murut, Kadazan and some African languages I do not know. I am lifted from depression, discouragement and despair as the prayers reverberate in my soul. I am grateful! I am humbled that you are praying!

Nothing has changed. The word "recovery" is not in the vocabulary of Alzheimer's. Devastation, delusion, destruction and disaster are all written into the disease. **But change is taking place!** Your prayers are opening the door of peace for me. Your prayers are sustaining Erica as she stumbles along the unknown path. Your prayers are giving me strength, patience, grace and understanding so I can, without ceasing, love her for you. I have more confidence as I face each unending day as we fumble our way through this disease. One husband walking this same pathway said, "It is not the mountains ahead of you that are the problem, but the grains of sand in your shoes day by day". Each day is another challenge. Each night is another emptiness. I am overcome with gratitude for your being there for us. The prayers of my interceding friends are the best and sometimes the only thing you can do.

Thank you for making it possible to walk this darkened way with the knowledge that I am not alone.

WAVES

MARCH 6, 2003

This morning as I was groping for a Rock of Scripture to stand on for this day I found firm footing on the miracle of Jesus walking on the water as recorded in Matthew 14:22-33; Mark 6:45-51 and John 6:16-21,

This week I have been, like the disciples, "straining at the oars". The wind and waves are against me. I feel I am making progress in discovering ways to help Erica then the wind and waves of Alzheimer's slaps me back. The disease is like the waves of the sea. It never stops. There are a few days when the waves gently nudge the shore of reality. There are days when the "surf is up" and it roars. It crashes! It froths and erodes! Shoved by a hurricane force it snaps all lines of communication. It crumbles old and dear foundations! It uproots sturdy trees of relationships! The undertow leaves me staggering and grasping to be able to stand— to be able to move forward. But the winds and waves are against me. They never stop. Incessantly they batter Erica and me. A dear friend, whose mother has Alzheimer's disease voiced it perfectly."This is the ugliest of diseases—it is the worst. It is like going through the grief process over and over again with no end in sight. Just as you begin to adjust to one part of losing them, and can rejoice in what is left, the process starts all over again". My friend, Dr. Wayne Ewing, who lost his wife to Alzheimer's before she was 60 years of age, said, "To be honest about my sense of loss. It is worse than death".

The last few days have been just that. The snarling wind and waves of the disease have snapped the line of being able to respond. The lines have become so corroded with dead and dying cells that there is no communication between eyes and ears and muscles. All lines are down. The arms and legs refuse to move or they do just the opposite of what is needed. She looks bewildered

31

when asked to lift a fork to eat or move her foot. There is no connection. Standing without assistance is impossible. The lines are crossed. Instead of standing the body becomes rigid –her arms stay folded in her lap---her feet won't cooperate. The waves of the disease have engulfed her in its fury. O, Lord, how do I save for a while what is left of my life sweetheart as she flounders in this frothy sea?

My doctors, my friends and the Alzheimer's organization all say, "Save the caregiver if you are to survive care giving". For me it must begin with Scripture, prayer and relationship to my Lord as I am *"buffeted by the waves because the wind was against it"* (Matthew 14:24). As I read over and over again this story I begin to see a crack of blue in the gray sky of distress. I am helped by the knowledge that there are others in the same boat (Mark 6:45). I am not alone in the restless sea. I am not alone in the struggle to survive and assist my loved one. Science and friends are striking the oars in harmony to deal with this disease. As age engulfs us more and more friends are encountering the disease in family or friends. I do not have to face the winds and waves alone. Jesus sees us "straining at the oars"(Mark 6:48.). He is getting in the boat with me (Mark 6:51). Jesus speaks words that are greater than the wind and waves. *"Take courage. It is I. Don't be afraid "(Mark 6:50) and "the wind died down"* (Matthew 14:32) His presence brings amazing peace. He words propel the boat toward the shore and they are safe and secure (John 6:21).

Reading this word I am moved to pray "O. Lord, please give me eyes to see you even through his stormy time. Don't let me be like the disciples who did not recognize You when You came to help. Make me a survivor. O, Lord, please let my faith be an anchor that is stronger than the waves and wind slamming Erica around and befogging her mind. Lord, do not let the undertow take away my ability to support her when she staggers and stumbles with this eroding disease. Daily remind me, *"For this God is our God forever and ever; He will be our guide even to the end" (Psalm 48:14).*

SHADOWS

MARCH 13, 2003

II went to bed with a heavy heart March 7. All night the shadowy images of Erica danced in and out of my dreams. I am so deeply concerned about her and how I can assist her in this unending battle against this most pervading disease. I awoke early to search my soul for answers. I was reliving the words of Aeschylus, the ancient Greek dramatist: *"Pain, that cannot forget, falls drop by drop upon the heart, until, against our will, and in our sleep, come wisdom, from the awesome grace of God."* Wisdom—I do not have but greedily seek. Grace of God—present and I hungrily seek more every day.

Erica wept last night as I was getting her ready for bed. She could not, or would not, tell me why. I wept with a feeling of helplessness. Getting her ready for bed is the most stressful time of the day. Why? She doesn't seem to understand the need to change from daytime to nighttime clothing. She resists the necessary bathroom activities. She seems unable to move her legs or hands or know what to do with them. She has difficulty standing or walking. I wept questioning, "Had I been impatient, unkind or rough with her in the process of getting her ready for bed?" I cuddled her and told her how much I loved her. She took my face in her hands and said, "I know you love me!" The pain of the moment ripped through my being. All night the dark shadow of that moment haunted my sleep. "O, Lord, I plead for wisdom. You promised *"For this God is our God for ever and ever; he will be our guide even to the end"*. (Psalm 48:14) I appeal to you to *"turn Your face toward me and give me peace"* (Numbers 6:24).

Shadows invade every aspect of life. At times they are just a momentary flicker. Other times they are deep and frightening. Real or imagined demons lurk in the shadows. Alzheimer's disease is a real demon. It is frightening! It has incapacitated Erica. A dear

33

friend wrote "It is frightening by the fact that this merciless disease lurks in the shadows, looking for more victims". Each day I hear of others who are being attacked by this insidious disease.

What to do? Defeat it? Impossible! Ignore it? Never! Face it? Yes, but not in my own strength! The world's best scientists and doctors have found it unconquerable. Families and friends weep and plead for relief but to no avail! The lengthening shadows of this debilitating disease invade every moment of every hour. There are times when *"My face is red with weeping, deep shadows ring my eyes" (Job 16:16)*. As I read Psalm 23 I was struck anew that everything in the psalm was positive. Even verse 4 *"Though I walk through the valley of the shadow of death, I will fear no evil, for you are with me, your rod and your staff, they comfort me"*. There are no shadows except there is a strong light behind the shadow. The promise was given *"on those living in the land of the shadow of death a light has dawned" (Matthew 4:16)*. John identifies that Light. Jesus spoke, *"I am the light of the world. Whoever follows me will never walk in darkness, but will have the Light of life" (8:12.)*.

There is Light and Life greater than the demon. I am promised, *"He reveals the deep things of darkness and brings deep shadows into the light" (Job 12:22)*. Daniel 2:20,22 praise the God of heaven as he writes, *"Praise be to the name of God forever and ever. He reveals deep and hidden things, he knows what lies in darkness, and light dwells with him"*. There is light at the end of the tunnel of Alzheimer's disease. *It is our Lord who promises "Never will I leave you, never will I forsake you" (Hebrews 13:5b)*.

There are good and bad shadows. Stressing only the bad, I miss the good. Isaiah 25 records, *"O Lord, you are my God. You are a refuge for the needy in distress, a shelter from the storm, and a shade from the heat—as heat is reduced by the shadow of a cloud—the Sovereign Lord will wipe away tears from all faces— surely this is our God; we trusted in him, and he saves us"*. Our

Lord provides that refreshing cloud and we must praise him and say, *"I will exalt you and praise your name" (verse 1).* In the stress and strain of every moment of each day the Lord reaches out and covers me with the shadow of His hand, saying, *"You are my people"* (Isaiah 51:16,17). This shadow allows me to go on ministering to my dear Erica, I am conscious of unusual strength, patience and peace under the shadow of His hand. I can pray and rejoice with David, *"Keep me as the apple of your eye; hide me in the shadow of your wings" (Psalm 17:8),* and know that there I am kept by His love for Erica and me. John Rohn, motivational speaker, said, "The walls we build around us to keep out sorrow also keep out joy". I must look for the strength and security from *"lying in green pastures";* and the restoration of soul that comes from *"quiet waters";* the Presence to *"guide me and comfort me"* and His *"goodness and love always" (Psalm 23).*

Erica's life has left its indelible mark on people in many states and foreign countries. The shadow of her incredible, positive spirit still springs vibrantly into many lives. The eroding disease may capture the bodily functions but it will never wipe out the greatness of her spirit and testimony. Her life changing contributions live on and on.

Victor Frankel, Austrian psychiatrist, who was imprisoned by the Nazis during the holocaust wrote "There is nothing in the world, I venture to say, that would so effectively help one to survive even the worst conditions as the knowledge that there is meaning in one's life". Erica's life has great meaning to family and friends of all races. I pray, "O Lord, help me make her remaining days a shining testimony of thy grace and meaningful to many in these days. May the shadow of her life make my days partially as meaningful as hers has been"..

WORRY

MARCH 15, 2003

One of the unwanted side effects of Alzheimer disease is "worry". Patients worry when they become aware of the loss of memory. They are concerned when they forget what they are doing, what they are saying, where they are going, where they have been and whom they have just seen. Worry is defined as "mental distress or agitation resulting from concerns, usually for something impending or anticipated". The family and especially the caregiver, experiences tautness in the stomach, disturbed sleep and invading concerns. They know the anticipated symptoms and they worry about when the next one is coming. They worry about how they will cope with the next development. Such has been this week.

Erica refuses to eat or seems to have forgotten how. Is this is the beginning of not being able to eat solid food? Is she going to start losing weight? Erica resists taking her medicine. Is this evidence that she is having difficulty swallowing? Erica sits and stares at me without saying a word. Is she slipping into failure to recognize who I am? At times she is not able to move her arms and legs. She has great trouble standing or walking. Her hands and legs shake unwittingly at times. Is this the first glimpse of immobility? Is this the beginning of inability to control the muscles? This is indeed a worrisome time. I worry about what is going to happen next. I worry if I will be able to cope with the next development. I know the symptoms of the various stages. I worry when the next one will appear.

Desperately looking for stability I plunge into God's word to discover how God related to worry. I was amazed that many translations do not use the word "worry". I did find "anxiety" and "fretting". Both are condemned and forbidden. Anxiety (as a noun) "is to be drawn in different directions". As a verb it "is to have a distracting care". The word "fret" means, "to blaze up" or "become warm".

Hungrily searching for answers I was led to Jesus' message on worry in Matthew 6:25-34. Four times Jesus spoke about the futility of being anxious (worry). He indicates that it is needless and useless. It will be injurious to my spiritual well being. Worry cannot change the past. Omar Khayyam grimly wrote--

"The moving finger writes, and having writ
moves on; nor all thy piety and wit
shall lure it back to cancel half a line,
nor all thy tears wash out a word of it".

Worry about the future is useless. Jesus said, *"Who of you by worrying can add a single hour to his life" (Matthew 6:27)*. I cannot alter the past to affect the future. He who provides for the birds and the things of nature will look after Erica and me because *"we are much more valuable than they" (verse 26)*. Paul reminds me *"My God will meet all your needs according to His glorious riches in Christ Jesus* (Philippians 4:19). William Barclay wrote "The lesson of life is that somehow we have been enabled to bear the unbearable and to do the undoable and to pass the breaking point and not to break".

Jesus reminds us that to worry is pagan (Matthew 6:32). It is lack of trust in God and His Word. Isaiah promises *"You will keep him in perfect peace him whose mind is steadfast, because he trusts in You" (26:3)*. "Lord, this is so easy to write, but so hard to do. Please, engrave on my mind and heart the way this can be. Grant me the faith! Give me the all-sufficient grace! Indelibly write them on my being! Let me learn afresh from You the way! Remind me that You care and are watching over Erica and me, even to knowing that *"The very hairs on your head are all numbered"* (Matthew 10:30).

Job reminds me to *"Submit to God and be at peace with Him (22:21)*. Jesus requested me to *"Seek first His kingdom and His*

37

righteousness, and all these things will be given to you as well" (Matthew 6:33). This is an invitation--yes, a command, to look above and beyond the problem and find the power to rise above worry. Paul wrote to the Corinthian, church *"I would like for you to be free from concern (worry)... (so) that you might live in a right way in undivided devotion to the Lord"* (1 Corinthians 7:32,25).

Worry becomes a sin and hinders the growth of peace in my mind and heart. I become one of those who *"though seeing, do not see; though hearing, do not hear or understand"* (Matthew 13:15). I am among those *who need to come to Him and "understand with their hearts and turn, and I would heal them" (Matthew 13:15).*

"O, Lord, give me *grace to follow your Word. Teach me again the game plan to victory over worry.* I ask for faith and grace to heed your word.

Psalm 57:1 - *"Have mercy on me, O God, have mercy on me, for in you my soul takes refuge. I will take refuge in the shadow of* thy wings until the disaster has passed." James 4:7-8,10 - *"Submit yourself to God. Resist the devil, and he will flee from you. Come near to God and he will come near to you. Humble yourself before the Lord, and He will lift you up".* I Peter 5:7, 10 *"Cast you all your anxiety (worries) on the Lord for he cares for you."* Psalm 55:22 - *"Cast your cares (worries) on the Lord and he will sustain you, he will never let the righteous fall".* Philippians 4:6,7 - Do *not be anxious about anything, but in everything, by prayer and petition, with thanksgiving, present your requests to God. And the peace of God, which transcends all understanding, will guard your heart and mind in Christ Jesus"*

"Thank you, Lord, for reminding me not to worry, but to trust, abide and be faithful to you. Lord, bless in your own way, all who are supporting Erica and me as we wander through this thicket of Alzheimer's disease".

FRIENDS

MARCH 22, 2003

Alzheimer's disease drives the patient, the family and the care-giver into a desert of frustration and despair. I identify with Psalm 63:1, which says, *"My soul thirsts for you, my body longs for you in a dry and weary land where there is no water"*. I feel like the bone thirsty deer that *"pants for streams of water"* (Psalm 42:1). Each morning I am driven into the desert to look for sustaining grace for me as I pray for directions for Erica's life and mine. My passion drives me like a prospector searching for gold. I know it is there, but where? Physical routines are followed. I search for ways to meet her emotional needs. She never complains. She ultimately will respond to what needs to be done. I am frustrated when she cannot form the words to communicate. I am wounded as I sense that my words or actions are complied with but not understood. Her mind cluttered with the debris of the disease, allows her to think she is complying but her body is doing the opposite. My soul is wrenched when I ask, "Do you understand?" and her beautiful brown eyes stare back at me and she remains mute. Oh, how I pray for an experience like John the Baptist when *"the word came to him in the desert"* (Luke 3:2).

As I eagerly dig for gold and a glimmer of hope it may be just a fleck of gold dust that glistens in the desert. It may be from the Scriptures, a devotional book or from your words to me. Sometimes it is a nugget of pure gold that sparkles in my soul. At time I strike the mother lode. The Word of God dazzles me with a profound hope and/or insight. An unexpected telephone call from Jakarta, Penang, Singapore or the U.S. inspires me. Email from you sharing a golden truth you have mined twinkles a truth into reality. My life is enriched by words from a song or poem you send. I cherish the panned gold that comes in unasked letters, visits or a choice item of food. Dear friends who come by to sit with Erica while I tend to business, go shopping or just give me a break enrich my life beyond words.

Alzheimer's disease rips apart the patient, the family and the caregiver. It also may cleave friendships. It may be the litmus test that strains friendships. Some with whom I thought I had welded unbreakable bonds have faded into a line in the address book. I may hear from them once a year when they send a printed Christmas card. Others who were just acquaintances have burst like a spring flower into a beautiful, caring, sustaining relationship. Walter Winch ell said, *"A friend is one who walks in when the rest of the world walks out. One who is here today and here tomorrow"*. My cherished psychiatrist friend explains it this way *"Some people do not trust their emotions enough to be meaningful involved with others in their pain and sorrow. They ignore the suffering, hoping it will go away. Some have wrapped themselves so tightly in their own life, desires and plans there is no crack that allows the concerns of others to enter"*. An anonymous writer wrote, *"Trouble is a big sieve through which we sift our acquaintances. Those who are too big to pass through are friends."*

Aristotle defined a friend as a "Single soul dwelling in two bodies". *Another calls it* "one heart in two bodies".

The New Testament uses two words for "friend". One is "comradeship". The other is one loved, —loving as well as being loved. An example of the depth of friendship is seen in these words *"the soul of Jonathan was knit with the soul of David, and Jonathan loved him as his own soul"* (I Samuel 18:1 KJV). When the disciples matured from thinking Jesus came only to deliver them from the Romans (Luke 24:21) to loving Him for who He was and what He would be to them Jesus called them "friends" (John 15:11-16). These friends He would love to the very end (John 13:1).

The difference between companions and friends is clarified in *"A man of many companions may come to ruin, but there is a friend*

40

who sticks closer than a brother" (Proverbs 18:24). Differences may arise but the strain never snaps the bonds of friendship. Jonathan expressed this to David *"Go in peace, for we have sworn friendship with each other in the name of the Lord, saying, 'The Lord is witness between you and me forever"* (1 Samuel 20:42).

What a friend we have in Jesus. Isaiah 54:10 reminds me ever day. *"Though the mountain be shaken and the hills be removed yet my unfailing love for your will not be shaken nor my covenant of peace be removed, says the Lord, who has compassion on you"*. Erica has been my best earthly friend for over 62 years. She will not wander alone in this desert of evil. I am assured that the Lord is with her. I am here for her until death parts us. I rejoice today in you! You have burst into our dilemma saying by word and deed "I am your friend! I am here! Don't fail to call" I am on my way to be beside you".

You have taught me much! I am by nature and upbringing a very independent person. Being cast into this desert I have learned that "no man is an island". If you are struggling with being a caregiver to a loved one let your friends be there for you. They are waiting.

TODAY AND TOMORROW

MARCH 29, 2003

The first two days of this week were good; The crocus surprised us as they peep out from their winter nap. Orchestras of Jonquils and Daffodils with their white and yellow trumpets are ready to bring us notes of joy. Like young ladies at their first prom the streets are filled with flowering trees. The pear tree dressed in virgin white intermingle with the delicate pink cherry blossoms and the large lavender magnolia blooms. The forsythia huddle together in shiny gold array. The budding trees are racing to see which will be the first to turn green.

Robins are jerking wiggling worms out of the ground for a tasty breakfast. The birds are harmonizing in the choir singing Hallelujahs to the Creator. The sun has kissed away the dullness of winter and all nature is rejoicing, Yes, it has been a great two days.

Erica has been more alert! She has gone for rides and walks to observe and praise the beauty around her. She has been more responsive. She is eating and enjoying her food. She is smiling and laughing. She is talking more. I am rejoicing!

Alzheimer disease is as fickle as a day in February; We are embraced with the warmth of the rays of the sun. Then the clouds tumble in. The wind whistles a dreary tune. Snow flakes flitter silently down and pile up. We shiver and bundle up. The sage says, *"Do not boast about tomorrow, for you do not know what a day may bring forth"* (Proverbs 27:1).

Last night the plaque of an Alzheimer winter returned. Erica is restless. She stares at me with pleading eyes. I hurry to her side. I cuddle her. I assure her. What? Why? How can I help? She is mute or mumbles words that are not understandable. I struggle to get her ready for bed. Her limbs don't want to move. I tuck her in. I cuddle her. I pray for her and me. I telephone our son. With his increasing knowledge of the disease he diplomatically assists but does not insist on any action. I tumble into bed to wrestle with dreams, thoughts and unsolved decisions. I join the prayer of the Psalmist. *"O Lord, the God who saves me, day and night. I cry out before you. May my prayer come before you; turn your, turn your ear to my cry* (Psalm 88:1,2). I hear James 4:13-17 warn, "Do not presume on tomorrow. Be sure your plans are as He wills." I hear Jesus advise, *"Each day has enough trouble of its own"* (Matthew 6:34). The Jewish proverb admonishes. *"Care not for the morrow. Perhaps you may not find tomorrow"*.

Over the kitchen table Erica posted these words –
>Yesterday is history,
>Tomorrow is a mystery,
>Today is a gift
>That is why it is called the Present.

The thought reminds me to trust *"Praise be to the Lord, our Savior who **daily** bears our burdens" (Psalm 68:19).* O Lord, Help me to trust. When I let worry obscure my sight, I miss so much.

Each morning I awaken Erica by singing Psalm 118:24 *"this is the day the Lord has made; let us rejoice and be glad in it"*. I tell her the time, the date and day. Then she opens her eyes and smiles at me. The tone of the day has been set. We are assured *"The day is yours, and yours also the night; you established the sun and moon. It was you who set all the boundaries of the earth; you made both summer and winter" (Psalm 74:16,17). It is His day!* I find my heart filled with confidence and joy that He is still in control even in the gnawing winter of Alzheimer's disease.

Psalm 139 is called "Prayer of the Presence". Walking through it my soul tingles with the excitement of knowing *"All the days ordained for me were written in your book before one of them came to be" (verse 16)*.

Numerous hospital stays, twelve surgeries and three life threatening experiences prompted me to print in large letters beside my office clock and over the kitchen table this reminder –

"One day at a time, and the day is His day;
He has numbered its hours, though they haste or delay,
His grace is sufficient; we walk not alone;
As the day, so the strength that He gives to His own".
--Annie Johnson Flint

I join in Wallace Fridy's prayer *"O God for another day, for another morning, for another hour, for another minute, for another chance to live and serve Thee, I am truly grateful. Do Thou this day free me from fear of the future; from anxiety of the morrow; for cowardice in the face of danger and from weakness when Thy power is at hand"*.

As I face the unknown future for Erica and myself I pray I will remember what God has *not promised* and what He has *promised so* eloquently written -

GOD HAS NOT PROMISED	GOD HAS PROMISED
Skies always blue,	Strength for the day,
Flower strewn pathways	Rest for the labor,
All our lives through;	Light for the ways,
God hath not promised	Grace for the trials
Sun without rain,	Help from above
Joy without sorrow	Unfailing sympathy
Peace without pain.	Undying love.

---Annie Johnson Flint

The future is cloudy. The forecast is for stormy days for Erica and me. No one can project the timing. I dare not presume how I will react from day to day as I try to secure the best care possible for her.

William Barclay said *"The true Christian way is not to be terrorized into fear, and not to be paralyzed into inaction by the uncertainty of the future, but to commit the future and all our plans into the hands of God and always to remember that our plans may not be within the purpose of God".*

So, I sing with Bill and Gloria Gaither—
> One day at a time, sweet Jesus
> That's all I am asking from you,
> Just give me the strength to do
> Everyday what I have to do.
> Yesterday's gone, sweet Jesus,
> And tomorrow may never be mine
> Lord, help me today, show me the way
> One day at a time

Lord, this is your day. Help me rejoice in the good days and trust in the days not so good. Help me to live this day to care for Erica the best I know, to trust in you for guidance and to help others who walk this same way.

DECISIONS

APRIL 4, 2003

It was 4:00 p.m. March 24, 2003. I foolishly thought I was prepared! I had prayed for strength and grace for this moment. The nurses knocked. They rolled Erica away. The click of the closing door burst the cisterns of my heart. I crumbled into the nearest chair. Hot tears breeched the dam of my eyelids and washed my face. My body shook with audible sobs. I wandered from room to room. Her side of the bed shrieked at me "She is not here!" Her favorite chair shouted at me "She is gone!" Her clothing rustled a hollow whisper, "You are alone!" My darling Erica, by doctor's orders, had been taken to the Alzheimer's Unit of the Health Care. Only five minute walk away. So near- yet so far. I wept as I had not done except when my mother was buried on May 26, 1970 (my birthday) and when our oldest son (named after me and born on my birthday died tragically July 21, 1992. I felt ripped apart. How long? Until there were no more tears to shed. Cold water lessened the heat of the tears but didn't relieve the ache. Doctors and nurses had advised, "This is best for her and you". Friends, who had walked this way ahead of me said, "We understand. It is best". Family assured me of support in the decision. **But, I had to make the decision.**

It has been said, "to not make a decision is to make a decision". The fracture caused by the decision would take much prayer before peace. would come.

April 3, 2003. Eleven days of agony my soul has wrestled with my decision. Each moment my thoughts are with her. Each night her empty bed haunts me. I need her! I want her here! I feel the voice of the Psalmist *"I am in pain and distress; may your salvation, O God, protect me (69:29).* I am struggling to be able to say *"I will praise God's name in song and glorify him with thanksgiving"* (Psalm 69:30).

46

For the first time I understand the emotional strain of following Jesus as recorded in Luke 9:57-62. For weeks I have listen (and shuttered) as Sid Reber sang the words written by Lanny and Marietta Wolfe.

"Take the dearest things to me, if that's how it must be
To draw closer to Thee;
Let the disappointments come, lonely days without the sun.
If thro' sorrow more like You I'll become!
That's what I'll be willing to do."

Within hours of notifying family and concerned friends I was flooded with telephone calls and emails from overseas and nearby with words of comfort, assurances of prayer support and love wrapping their arms around me. I felt lifted up on the wings of prayer. My hatred was riveted against the disease that had captured my dearest. It separated us for the first time in over 60 years. Question? Do I allow hatred for something I cannot control to consume me to the point I will not honor Christ and not be able to help others? I was alone – yet not alone! I was reminded that Jesus *"always lives to intercede for me"* (Hebrews 7:25). Your prayers began to mold my being. Strength flowed in and engulfed my weakness. I was aware that I not only was praying to God but praying with God and others. I was experiencing Ecclesiastes 4:9-12 *"Two are better than one—If one falls down, his friend can help him up. A cord of three strands is not quickly broken"*.

How did I arrive at this heart-breaking decision? I stand in an ever-increasing crowd, *"Multitudes, multitudes in the valley of decision! The earth and sky will tremble but the Lord will be a refuge for his people"* (Joel 3:14-16). With clearer eyes meaning leaped from the sign Erica posted over the dining table *"Do not feel totally, personally, irrevocably responsible for everything. This is my job! Love, God"*.

One decision demands making more decision. In my role as minister of pastoral care, I had walked quickly by the Alzheimer's unit On first furtive glance it is not very conducive to lingering. Souls, with befogged minds are at all levels of senility, dementia and Alzheimer's. None chose to be here. All would escape if they could. Now, I must see them differently. Erica is one of them. I must take notice and appreciate the loving care the attendants are giving them.

I processed this decision for several months. Several things had to take place before I gained the consent of my soul to make the hardest decision I have ever had to make. Even as I write these words I ache and tears flow. The adjustment is like a dreadful nightmare that does not want to end.

I hear the words of Elijah *"How long will you waver between two opinions? If the Lord is God—follow Him"* (I Kings 18:21). Erica's condition was declining daily. I did not want to admit I no longer could give her the physical care she needed. What is best for Erica? Where will she receive the care she needs? I was frustrated, very tired and becoming impatient with myself, with Erica and my continuing ministry to others. I must make a decision. The decision had to be **decisive**. How would I arrive at the point of decision?

Decision must be based on **discernment**. I must have *peace with the decision.* Assurance flooded in *"My soul finds **rest** in God alone; One thing God has spoken, two things I have heard: that you, O God, are strong, and that you, O Lord, are loving"* (Psalm 62:1,11,12). Psalm 139:5,7 reassured me. No matter where I, or Erica, may be, God is with us. God can take better care of her than I because *"he who watched over you will not slumber, Indeed, he will neither slumber or sleep"* (Psalm 121:3,4). My mind reeled but a quiet, gentle breeze of peace began to sweep over my soul and I was refreshed.

My decision must be based on **knowledge.** I sought wisdom from those who had been there before me. I inquired about care, conditions, food and attitudes. I must have **confidence**. in the nurses, social welfare staff and aides. I had to feel secure in entrusting my most precious person to others.

For over two years I had been enveloped in a cloud of doubt. I was afraid for Erica and myself. I needed to hear the words, *"When my heart was grieved and my spirit embittered, I was senseless and ignorant; Yet I am always with You; You hold me by my right hand. You guide me with your counsel"* (Psalm 73:21-23). Wonderfully, the cloud lifted. A shaft of peace pierced my inner most being.

Decision must have **determination**. I could not waver! Three days after Erica moved she said to me *"this is my home now"*. I was crushed. I choked on my words. For over 60 years wherever we were it was "our" home. Now it is "my home". I was not beside her. Each night as I cuddle her, pray with her and tell her how much I love her she says "please, don't leave me". I rapidly walk away so my tears will not reveal how badly I hurt. It has to be this way. We wouldn't choose it. The despicable disease forced it upon us.

Erica is in "her" home and I in my lonely apartment. What now? She will ever remain my number one human priority! She is first in my continuing ministry to others.

I will visit her several times a day.

I will carry some of my meals and eat with her in her room.

I will cuddle her and assure her of my love several times a day.

I will bring her small gifts I know she likes.

I will encourage her friends to visit her, send picture cards and letters.

(She holds them in her hand and reads them over and over).

I will still be her caregiver. I will. provide her needs and wants.

I will not allow her to be forgotten. Her cluttered mind may forget but her story will not be unwritten.

I will minister to her fellow residents and to others as Jesus
told me
"As you did for one of the least of mine, you did for me"
(Matthew 25:40).

If you know one who is imprisoned by this relentless disease do
not forget them. Do not fail to love them. Keep them in your life.
They are still a worthwhile person with dignity. Remember who
they were and rejoice in what they still are. You may not have
another chance.

IMPRISONMENT

APRIL 11, 2003

Alzheimer's disease is very much like being in prison. The bleak walls of hopelessness press in on every side. This morning Proverbs 12:25 spoke to me, *"An anxious heart weighs a man down, but a kind word cheer him up"* Friends fulfill the saying "I believe that friends are quiet angels who lift us to our feet when our wings have trouble remembering how to fly".

Alzheimer's disease is like riding a roller coaster. There are days when Erica is up--articulate, responsive and adjusting well. Just when she and I are shrieking for joy and delighting in this we are hurtled back into reality. She is confused! My stomach is churning and roiling! I am hurting! She wants me there all the time. Recently I had to attend to some business. A dear friend was with her. Erica kept peeking out the door. The friend asked "Are you hungry". Erica replied, "Yes, I am hungry for my husband". When I was told this a bullet of guilt ricocheted through me ripping open the wound of separation. What to do? As bedtime approaches each night she become restless and keeps looking at the door. She senses the attendant is coming to prepare her for bed. When she does come, Erica turns those beautiful brown eyes toward me and pleads, "don't leave me".

With mind reeling, I make my way to the apartment. As I open the door a blast of loneliness rumbles out followed by a flash of silence. At night I find myself awakening and looking for the familiar bump of her body. I reach out my hand to touch her and shudder as I find only the cold pillow.

Erica and I are imprisoned. Nothing we did brought on this crippling disease, but we are imprisoned by it. Alzheimer is the Alcatraz of diseases. It is the worst of the worst. Its' fangs have sunk deep into Erica's brain and poisoned the intellect, creativity, comprehension and abilities of my dearest friend. There is no known antidote. She is imprisoned. There are no bars on the windows. There is no restriction of movement. No guards shuffle up and down the corridor. There are no limits placed on visitation. Yet she is imprisoned. The disease has locked securely her ability to read with comprehension, to write or to function in most matters. The familiar is becoming unfamiliar,

At times she is placed in the confinement of silence. She is sentenced to be confined at the will of the disease. The gray walls of Erica's mind imprison her from friends, her intimate relationships, normal life style and me. The impregnable bars shut out the joys and partnership of 62 years of very happy life together. She is physically well. Yet this ruthless disease shackles the most vital part of her. Her mind has been sentenced to death's row from which there is no pardon. My heart wrenches as she struggles to speak and her vocabulary has been reduced to just pointing. I agonize to try to find meaning to what she wants or needs.

I also am imprisoned for the duration. I am committed to her "till death do us part". Where do I turn? There are times I am like David in the cave of En Gedi imprisoned by fear of what Saul would do to him (1 Samuel 24:1,3). While hiding there David wrote Psalm 142. *"I cry aloud to the Lord. I lift up my voice to the Lord of mercy. Listen to my cry for I am in desperate need. When my spirit grows faint within me, I cry to you, O Lord, you are my refuge. Set me free from my prison, that I may praise your name because of your goodness to me"* (1,6,3,5,7). I join J.W. Whittier in praying
> "Drop the still dew of quietness
> Till all our strivings cease;
> Take from our souls the strain and stress,
> And let our ordered lives confess
> The beauty of thy peace".

My imprisoned soul has been encouraged by Jesus' proclamation *"The Spirit of the Lord is upon me-He has sent me to proclaim freedom for the prisoners-to release the oppressed"* (Luke 4:18).

Today I turned to Paul's imprisonment in Philippians. The statement, *"I have learned to be content"* shocks me. *"I have learned the secret of being content in any and every situation"* (Verses 11,13). How Paul? How? *"I can do everything through him who gives me strength"* (verse 13).

The word "content" means "to have sufficient strength in oneself". Tell me, Paul, how do I reach that state of contentment? The strength is found in verses 4-10. There is to be *"rejoicing in the Lord always"* (v. 4).

I count my blessings. I remember how the Lord has privileged Erica and me to serve Him in ministry in many places in the world. There is much to rejoice in. There is to be an obvious, accepting attitude of faith and trust (Philippians 1:12-14).

Richard Niebuhr prayed-
> "God grant me the serenity
> To accept the things I cannot change
> Courage to change the things I can
> And wisdom to know the difference".

There is to be prayer with thanksgiving, bringing the peace of God, which transcends all understanding. There must be determination to center my thoughts on the goodness of God and not on the disease gnawing at the brain of Erica and attempting to stifle my soul. I pray, "Lord, do not let me forget *'How precious to me are your thoughts, O God! How many are the sum of them! Were I to count them, they would out number the grains of sand"*. (Psalm 139:17,18.

While Alzheimer's disease erodes the mind of Erica it cannot imprison her soul. She will not fade into nothingness. Many letters, calls and friends are even now recognizing her life, smile, testimony and ministry. As for me I pray "Let not my anxious thoughts be an offense to you and give me strength for each day. Grant me freedom in my soul even in my imprisonment".

GUILT

APRIL 18, 2003

This is Holy Week. I am seeing it through the eyes of a caregiver for my precious wife. The agony of watching Erica struggle with this corroding disease is sparking all kinds of feelings. I remember the triumphs of her life and ministry. Memories of her sacrifice in caring for me through two heart surgeries, ear surgery, cancer and chemotherapy flood my mind.

I rejoice in the great joy of her 83rd birthday celebrated on April 12. Her room was strewn with over 125 cards, letters and email. Chocolates and flowers were abundant. Eric, our son, flew in from New York City for the day. She was happy, responsive and talking. She chose the food she wanted to eat and ate it with gusto. In the midst of triumph the threatening clouds began to roll in. I reached out to her but she was unresponsive. She was marching to the demands of the angry disease. I could only watch and hurt. A flash of guilt burned its way into my entire being. I had shared with her such a beautiful life dedicated wholly to God and committed to sacrificial service to others in the U.S., Singapore, Malaysia, Philippines and Borneo. Remembering her talents and ministry was such a joy.

As I watched her sink into the fog of forgetfulness, apprehension grabs at my soul. My bed is rumpled up from tossing and turning in agony. My thoughts are twisted and direction is unclear. A finger of guilt jabs at my heart. How am I to handle this pain of guilt? Questions wash over me. Have I broken my wedding vows to take care of her "for better or worse—in sickness and in health?" Did I fail her by not seeing the creeping disease soon enough and get her treatment and medication? Am I doing right by continuing my ministry to the church and others and not being with her as much as she wants? Am I selfish in returning to the apartment when she begs me not to leave her alone in the Health Care room? Am I washing my hands of her by not keeping her at home?

The demon of guilt is having a good time with me. I an ensnared! I search for the trigger to release me from the steely spikes of the trap of guilt and find total and constant peace. What am I to do?

I flip the pages of my Bible. The fiery words of Jesus leap from a page *"Men should always pray and **not give up**"* (Luke 18:1). The challenge of the parable is that in order for me to receive the relief I seek, I must be found as a man of faith.

The word "guilt" means "to be held in a fixed position or to be ensnared". Alzheimer's has trapped Erica. It is not possible to open the jaws of the trap. No scientific or medical knowledge can free her. The disease cannot conquer her soul but only shackle her mental functions. Am I hindering her if I allow guilt to entrap me? At present I jerk at the chain of the trap but am not free. Am I dishonoring my Lord and crippling my ministry to Him, Erica and others by being entrapped with guilt?

I put my soul under the microscope of God's Word and search for guidance. I Corinthians 10:13 challenges me, *"No temptation has seized you except what is common to man. And God is faithful; he will not let you to be tempted beyond what you can bear. But when you are tempted, he will also provide a way out so that you can stand up under it".* No temptation can seize me if I avoid walking into the trap.

Feelings of guilt can entrap me only if I allow myself to wander where it lies waiting. The Lord brought Psalm 84:6,7 to my attention. The valley of Baca is a figurative description of the "valley of weeping." The salty drops of tears turn into refreshing springs and all sufficient pools of joy as *"they go from strength to strength".* I gulp down Psalm 85:8, *"I will listen to what God the Lord will say; he promises peace to his people, his saints—but let them not return to folly".* The peace I seek is to be found in not returning to the folly of guilt. How to escape the hidden trap of guilt that awaits me?

I am grateful and indebted to my cherished friend and Greek scholar, Johnnie Godwin, for his guidance in my understanding of Philippians 4:13: The word "through" should be translated "in" He lovingly admonished me "You can't do everything. You can't do all things through Christ. But you can do everything He wants you to do in the sphere of His will. And I believe you're doing that right now ". This breath of fresh air helped scatter the cloud of guilt.

He further reminded me that Easter always follow Good Friday. by referring to 2 Corinthians 4:14-5:10 *"Therefore we do not lose heart. Though outwardly we are wasting away, yet inwardly we are being renewed day by day"* (4:16,17). He identifies with the struggle as he watches his mother with the same horrendous disease as Erica. His final remarks are good for me to treasure. "God has a better experience for us ahead. The best may have been on earth, and the worst may be ahead; but the best of all is still to come. That's the message of Easter".

Erica and others wandering in the fog of the disease will have a renewal of mind and a body greater than ever known on earth. Christ will break the chains of the debilitating trap and Erica will be free.

I must be free from the trap of guilt if I am to be a helpful caregiver to Erica and to others, I must be alert that guilt does not sneak up on me. Proverbs 11:24,25 must be remembered *"One man gives freely, yet gains even more; a generous man will prosper; he who refreshed others will himself be refreshed."* It is what we give and not what we receive which produces joy and happiness. As the anonymous poet said—

> Not what we have, but what we give
> Not what we see, but how we live—
> These are the things that build and bless
> That lead to human happiness.

My prayer to escape the snares of the "guilt trap" must be *"Teach me your way, O Lord, and I will walk in your truth; give me an undivided heart, that I may fear your name. I will praise you, O Lord my God, with all my heart; I will glorify your name forever. For great is your love toward me; you have delivered me from the depth of the grave (guilt)".*

BANKRUPTCY AND RECOVERY

APRIL 25, 2003

Alzheimer's disease makes me poorer each day. The insidious disease continues to nibble away at Erica and in doing so erodes me emotionally. This past week I have been teetering on the edge of emotional bankruptcy. Erica's 83rd birthday was a deposit of great happiness. Eric, our son, was here and she enjoyed the attention, flowers, cake, and good meals. When I showed her the pictures of the events there was a huge withdrawal. She looked at each picture for hours. She recognized Eric and me. Pointing at herself she asked, "Who is this woman?" My emotional balance was sent quivering. Was she losing her self-identity?

Being notified that two articles of mine had been accepted for publication by the *Mature Living* magazine was a silver lining to a dark cloud. Sorrow gripped me when I remembered that since my first book was published in 1956 and seven other books and numerous articles, this was the first time I was denied the partnership of Erica in them. She had always been my confidant, my constructive critic, contributor, editor and encourager. Each idea had been examined under the microscope of her superior ability in language, syntax, grammar and content. Her spiritual sensitivity pierced through every word of each sentences pointing out misused words, construction, usage and clarity. Alzheimer's has short-circuited the hum of her mental processing. Her wise eyes are blurred to the textual inconsistencies. How I ache to hear her say, "This could be said in a better way". I long to hear her helpfully criticize the contents. I need to hear her say, "This is good. You have done well. I rejoice in your gift of writing".

She hears me speak but is unmoved. The wreath of victorious acceptance wilts without her understanding and approval. Her helpfulness to me is restricted and I am left poverty stricken.

Now she mumbles, "Whatever you think". I hate those words. The disease pilfers my life. I want her input and advice as I write her life story. She has been told I am doing it but can't contribute to make it more authentic and inspiring. It will be written but it will not be as inspiring as if she were able to partner with me.

Sunday worship services nudged me closer to bankruptcy. After my part in the service I always sat beside her. As I sat down she would squeeze my hand and say a sweet word. Yesterday I sat down where we usually sat. Unconsciously my hand reached for hers. It wasn't there. No word of encouragement was said. I shivered and hit the bottom emotionally. I fought the urge to leave the service. I am so poor without her presence.

It is night. The black veil of loneliness is all around me. It is time for me to balance my emotional books. Reflecting I discover deposits had been made to my account. My pastor had made a deposit when he quoted 1 John 1:4, *"Our fellowship is with the Father and with the Son, Jesus Christ—this is to make our joy complete"*. Disease cannot corrupt that joy and fellowship. I am enriched.

After service several expressed love and concern for Erica and me. One lovely lady, noting my condition, said

"We need you here. You are helping so many of us as we face our problems". Ecclesiastes 4:9,10,12 clamored for my attention *"Two are better than one, because they have a good return from their work. If one falls down, his friend can help him up. Though one may be overpowered, two can defend themselves"*.

Another deposit slip numbered 1 John 1:7 *"If we walk in the light, we have fellowship with one another"*. The balance looks better.

A missionary friend, whom I had not heard from for years, sent a deposit. Paraphrasing Philippians 1:7 "you have a special place." The card quoted the poem by Perry Tanksley—

"God said, "Go on! Don't quit!
Your work is not in vain.
I will always go with you
To strengthen and sustain."

I said, "God, I'm convinced
That I don't walk alone,
But there are days when I
Lack courage to go on".

God said, "Go on! Don't quit!
Remember, I love you,
Victory is just ahead
And I will see you through".

I was walking with Erica. We were greeted by a warm kiss from the sun. The yellow and white Iris lilies wave a welcome for us to sit on a bench in their midst. Erica leaned over and put her head on my shoulder. She whispered, *"I am so happy I have you. You take such good care of me"*. This was the biggest deposit of the day. Books closed! The deposits of God's Word, the presence of Christ, the fellowship of friends and Erica's love closed the day with a hefty balance.

Emotionally the battle against the disease will continue. My prayer is that these deposits will continue to bear interest and mature with great enrichment of my life and through me the lives of others who battle the same enemy.

DISRUPTION

MAY 2, 2003

Caregivers are perpetually suffering loss. Loss, that is not called for, or the result of any action on their part. Alzheimer's brings loss to everyone and it comes to stay. Every person either is, has been, will be or be in need of a caregiver. Alzheimer's winds sweep into homes and create disruption. The word "disrupt" means "to break apart or throw into disorder". The degenerative disease disrupts happy homes. Reaction to the effects of the disease is what is important. Jesus taught this lesson in John 9:1-3. We cannot undo the effects of Alzheimer's disease but we can show *"the work of God might be displayed in his life"* (verse 3).

A happy home is glued together by the commitment to each other. Sharing, like a rubber band, stretches to meet problems and sorrows and relaxes to bring joys.

As Erica and I reached retirement we felt secure. We had no debts. Our car was relatively new and paid for. We had a beautiful apartment in a wonderful retirement home. We had 24 hours security and medical care. The staff at the home was dedicated to meet our needs. Our apartment was alive with memories of family pictures and inspiring reminders of our ministries. Our children were well educated and happy in their chosen careers. We had sufficient funds to meet our needs and to come and go as we pleased. We were accountable to no one except the Lord and each other. For our age, we were in reasonable good health. Our cup was running over with happiness.

Like a bolt of lightening Alzheimer's disease reared its grotesque head and began to gnaw away at Erica's mind. Our happy home is disrupted. Our peaceful world began to spin out of control. Everything is topsy-turvy. Plans were shoved aside or put on indefinite hold. Shared chores now become my daily responsibility. My ministry is cut back and Erica's ground to a screeching halt. My life style of being highly organized and orderly is shoved aside. Meeting Erica's needs meant dropping everything and running to her side. Her several needs became domineering requirements. No matter how involved I was I stopped immediately to try to meet her needs.

When she could not voice the words I tried to interpret her actions. Frustrated? Yes! If she wanted to walk—we walked. If she needed bathroom attention, it was immediately cared for. If she wanted to go for a drive, I drove at once. My well-organized life began to come unglued. Our happy home now is two separate rooms. Only five minutes walking in the same building, but worlds apart. Our inspiring times of sharing are now one sided. Plans are altered each day. Dreams are in shambles, Alzheimer's is the cruel taskmaster disrupting everything. We are bound by the NOW. Hope is muddled. My desires are all squashed beneath my efforts to minister to her. A sudden change in the rampaging Alzheimer's calls for immediate alteration.

In the prayer of an afflicted man (Psalm 102) David wrote, *"I have become like a bird alone on a roof. All day long my enemy (Alzheimer's) taunts me" (verses 7,8).*

I am reminded, *"God is not a God of disorder but of peace"* (I Corinthians 14:33). Is it possible to have peace in this disorder? Is it possible to have hope in the midst of hopeless disruption? Jesus said it was! *"Peace I leave with you, my peace I give you. I do not give to you as the world gives. Do not let your hearts be troubled and do not be afraid."* (John 14:37).

I ache for the days past. I want to wipe away the fog. I want us to sit and share together. I long to hear her pray for others and me. I want to ease her troubled spirit. I want to reminiscence with her about the past and plan for the future. Alzheimer's has built a wall, which I cannot scale. The nurse and aids are doing a wonderful ministry in attention and medically caring for Erica and me. But this is not enough to remove the disruptions. What must I do? My soul quivers as I hear the answer. *"The Counselor, the Holy Spirit, whom the Father will send in my name, he will remind you of everything I have said to you"* (John 14:26). *The* Counselor (the Holy Spirit) is the God-provided Person who can be called to my side or aid. The touch of the Divine is available. Jesus promises *"I will not leave you as orphans. I will give you the Counselor to be with you forever—the Spirit of truth. He lives within you and will be with you"* (John 14:16-18).

"O Lord, Erica and I cannot have what we once enjoyed. We cannot live as we had anticipated. Help me not to be a worrier restating my present and anticipated worries. Move my petitions beyond gloomy desperation. Help me embrace with hope and expectation, *"God is able to do exceedingly abundantly above all we ask or think"* (Ephesians 3:20). Empower me to live beyond the unchangeable circumstances of Alzheimer's and by your grace walk with confidence in God and with His peace in my heart".

CLOCK WATCHING

MAY 28, 2003

I am a "clock watcher"! The clock over my desk ticks relentlessly. It is a hard task master drumming out the time to do something for Erica. When she was in the apartment her every movement was a command to meet her need. She is now in very capable and caring hands in the Health Care Unit. No matter where I am my mind runs back and forth to her room. My eyes are glancing at the watch or clock. Is it time for me to go to be with her? What is she doing now? Is she lonely or active? Is she alert? Is she eating and drinking sufficiently? Nancy L. Mace and Peter V. Rabins wrote an excellent guide for caregivers to a person who has Alzheimer's disease. The title, *The 36 Hour Day*, is not an exaggeration. The caregiver is chained to the clock to give care to a loved one. It is insistent and continuous! It is frustrating and tiring! I have complete confidence in the loving persons who are caring for Erica. They are more than just someone to look after Erica's needs.

Helen Keller wrote *"What we have enjoyed we can never lose. All that we have loved deeply becomes a part of us"*. Everything I am or ever wanted to be has been ripped out of my life. Life is disjointed! I am as frazzled as a worn out shirt collar. I have not lost her physically. She is here but she isn't. Emotionally and mentally the horrific disease has robbed her of identity. No longer is she able to contribute meaningfully to my life. She no longer is a supporting partner in the ministry, which we so enjoyed together for over 61 years. Each tick of the clock is a hollow reminder of hours enjoyed in the past and a frightening reminder of the hours to come.

Where is the "key" to unlock the handcuffs that chain me to the clock? What are the differences between minutes, hours, days and what time really should be?

Henry Wadsworth Longfellow wrote—
"The shadow on the dial,
The striking of a clock,
Those are but arbitrary and outward signs,
The measure of TIME but not TIME itself.
TIME is the life of the soul."

Samuel Liptzen said, *"A clock is a devise which owns no more than sixty minutes an hour"*. Edmund Rowland Sill defined the way life should be-
"Make the forenoon sublime
The afternoon a psalm
The night a prayer
And TIME is conquered and thy crown is won".

Ecclesiastes speaks ten times of activities as "chasing after the wind" and declared them "meaningless" causing days to be filled with pain and grief, even at night the mind does not rest (2:23). After observing "everything done under the sun (1:11) he concludes *"There is a time for everything, and a season for every activity under heaven" (3:1)*. The word "hour" in both Greek and Hebrew refers to "an indefinite period of time".

Seven couplets are listed in Ecclesiastes3: 1-8 with each one expressing two opposite reactions. He says, *"this is a gift of God so that men will revere Him"(3:13,14). "He has made everything beautiful in its time"* (3:11). God has given to man a sense of time so that there *"is nothing better for men than to be happy and do good while they live"* (3:12). There is an alternative for every "time" The clock does not measure life! It shows I have alternatives as to what I do with the moments and hours I have. Paul warned us *"Be careful how you live—not as unwise but as wise, making the most of every opportunity, because the days are evil"* (Ephesians 5:16,17).

After weeks of wrestling with this concern, I have discovered that *"a heart at peace gives life to the body"* (Proverbs 14:30). Time must be evaluated on the plan and purpose of God. *"I was pushed back and about to fall, but the Lord helped me. The Lord is my strength and my song; He has become my salvation. I will not die but live, and will proclaim what the Lord has done"* (Psalm 118:13,14,17).

Amy Carmichael, a missionary who knew much pain and suffering wrote, *"In acceptance lies peace"*. Horatius Bonar put it this way—

> "My times are in your hands,
> My God I wish them there.
> My life, my friends, and my soul- I leave
> Entirely in your care"

Another missionary wrote. "God sees and acts so as to meet the needs of the moment".

I reflect with gratitude in, *"Be at rest once more, O my soul, for the Lord has been good to you"* (Psalm 116:7).

I still have TIME! I still have LIFE! Erica and I did not cause this disease. We can't change or cure it. It must not rob us of the good there is while we still have time. Time must be appreciated not appraised.

I wheeled Erica into the beautiful rose garden. My eyes filled with tears of joy as she tenderly caressed the roses and admired their beauty. I thought, "This is wonderful. She is doing o.k.". In a few minutes the disease had slammed shut the sights of beauty and she was back into an unreal world". O, Lord, how this hurts! Please work your grace in me and help me to accept what I cannot change. Help me to rejoice in the times when she is alert and enjoying beauty and people. Time must be quality not quantity.

The clock still clamors for me to be with her—to help her take her meals—to sit quietly holding her hand—to walk beside her and keep her from stumbling. She is alert to my presence. She does well when I am not there. My emotional needs can't be met by the hours we are together but what we experience when we are together. Time must be a choice not a chore.

I must quit "beating the clock". My rushing through ministry, luncheons, and/or services so I can return to her only brings frustration, I can't regulate the stress of this heinous disease but I can control my reactions to it as far as time is concerned. Ministry to others will ignite compassion and strengthen me to be a better caregiver to Erica.

COMMUNICATION

JUNE 20, 2003

You don't miss communicating until you can't do it! Stimulating dialogue, inspiring suggestions, creative criticism and loving words were a vital part of my life with Erica. Since she was a Christian before I ever heard about Christ, she taught me words I needed to know. She led our prayer life. She initiated or helped develop the plans of our ministry. She was a strong vocal mentor to me and to hundreds in the U.S. Malaysia, Singapore, Borneo and the Philippine Islands. Her quiet voice spoke volumes. When she spoke silence fell like a curtain so her words could be heard.

The book of Proverbs defines communication being "choice silver" (10:20), "nourishing" (10:21), "bringing forth wisdom" (10:31), "healing" (11:19), "commanding knowledge" (15:2), "turning away wrath" (15:1), "apples of gold in a setting of silver and an ornament of fine gold" (25:11,12) and is "the law of kindness" (31:26). All this, and more, Erica was to me, her family, friends and all who crossed her life. How confused and empty is my life since Alzheimer's disease installed the bridle of silence. The disease has reined in her ability to speak as she once did. Her words are few and mostly disjointed. Seldom can she chain words together into much of a sentence. When she does speak, it is slow and low. My whole being aches as I strain to communicate with her. I am frustrated. She either does not respond or does not seem to understand. What to do? I must communicate with her! I am learning several things that help me.

RESPECT. No one knows what she understands. She is still a very dignified lady. She still notices little things. Her skills of communication are much like a child, but I will not treat her like a child. She is an adult. I will not demean her by using baby talk. I will not fuss about her inability to speak I will praise her for what she is able to do.

PRESENCE. Erica brightens up when I appear, She may not speak, but she knows I am there. I make her feel special and assure her of my love. I kiss her in front of the nurses and aids. I want them to know she is special and I will be there for her. Being with her every day is a priority.

PRESENTATION. Erica lives in the here and now. I try to move into her world and find her. The skill of remembering has been disrupted. I assure her who I am. When visitors come I introduce them to her. If Jesus felt it necessary to introduce Himself more than 20 times to confused and hurting persons how much more do I need to remind her who I and others are. This week I showed her an old photo album. She laughed at the picture of herself and her family. Alzheimer's patients can easily become confused. The thought process is all tangled up. I don't need to add to the confusion by playing guessing games with her. I do not ask her "why" or "who" or open-ended questions. I face her and speak calmly and quietly to her in short simple words. When I ask her too much or of I ask her to make decisions between two or more things she respond, "I don't know". I give the most important words at the end of a conversation and requiring only a "yes" or "no" reply.

PATIENCE.. At time Erica doesn't know how to respond. Her ability to sort through information takes time. By the time she has reached a comprehension she may have forgotten the subject. I give time for the information to worm its way through the tangled nerves. I often will repeat or even drop the subject or information, I tell her what I have been doing and the news. I read to her the greeting and prayer cards she has received. When she does respond, I listen carefully and respond with full attention. The other night I was delayed by over an hour from being with her when I usually am. I do not know that she knew this, but it bothered me greatly because I want to be with her and I did not want her to feel my delay as being neglect. I took her face in my hands and apologized for being late. I assure her of my love and my desire to be with her. I waited for her response. She understood. She reached up with her hand and stroked my face. This brought tears of joy to my eyes and I could not speak for a few minutes. This fulfilled for me Ecclesiastes 7:8: *"The end of a matter is better that the beginning, and patience is better than pride"*.

My prayer is I will develop more of the fruit of the Spirit "patience" (Galatians 5:22).

TOUCHING. Erica is not what she was mentally but she is still the wonderful, sweet person she always was. Her smile is just as spontaneous and beautiful as ever. She responds with a beautiful smile when I smile at her. I use the same endearing names with her. She is not an "it"! I intend for her to feel my touch. Touching is important! Jesus "touched" hurting people and blessings flowed from Him to them. It is no less with Erica. I kiss her often. I touch her hair. I pat her. She may or may not respond outwardly but I want her to feel the great love I have for her. Many times we communicate in silence as we hold hands. When she seems to have wandered away from me I will use my touch to bring her back to the now.

BODY LANGUAGE. The eyes, hands, body movements all have a voice. Erica may not speak in audible terms but her body communicates tremendous messages. At times she cannot verbalize her needs but she communicates with her body. When the body speaks it has my full attention. Loving her as I do, I watch her every movement when I am with her. I am quick to respond and try to interpret her needs. It takes patience and alertness to understand but I am learning.

Communication is essential in every relationship. It becomes more difficult with an Alzheimer's patient. I cannot and will not be robbed of communicating with Erica. It is not as it once was. I am told it will become more difficult, but I will still communicate with her. Erica will never be beyond my efforts to

70

communicate my love and admiration for her, My daily prayer is *"The Sovereign Lord has given me an instructed tongue to know the word that sustain the weary"*(Isaiah 50:4). To Erica I want to be like Job *"who strengthened feeble hands. Your words have supported those who stumbled; you have strengthened faltering knees"*(Job 4:3,4).

MEMORIES

JULY 26, 2003

God admonishes many times in the Scriptures *"Remember and don't forget"*. 2 Peter 1:13-15 challenges: *"I think it is right to refresh your memory"* and encourages us to *"always be able to remember"*. God created man with an unlimited memory bank. Memory causes bursts of laughter and joy. At times memory floods in with a surging ache or hot tears. Memory is always present unless the brain is damaged beyond the ability to recall,

As I began to put pen to paper to write the next chapter in the life story of Erica I was jolted with the thought *"this is no longer **her** story it is now **our** story"*. I am now a part of the rest of her life.

Researching her roots has been an adventure. To see history unfold her life like a hand fan has been exciting. Little nuggets of gold dripped out of every crevice of her life. What a thrill to see God mold this beautiful, wonderful life. Watching God weave into her life influences that produced a call to become a devoted servant of God has been exhilarating

The next chapter of her life is not history. It is reality! The door of the present is flung open. The files of memory are clicked "open". Each moment, each event, each word blazes out a memory. This has been bittersweet. Memory is either joy and happiness or regrets and tears. Not so for Erica. Alzheimer's has corroded her brain nerves. She feels little or nothing. Her emotions appear deadened. I cannot chisel my way into her memory. Her response to me is cold. Holding hands has always been our sweet connection. We have walked with tightly gripped hands in jungles, lakefronts, seasides, and snowy paths. We have held hands in ministry experiences and in bed. Now this act of sweet communion seems to be wrapped in a bundle and tightly tied with a string of *"I don't remember"*. *Like* a dagger these words cut into my soul. Rarely does the disease loosen to respond. Faces of loved ones usually bring a blank stare. Thrilling experiences cannot be recalled. Pictures of the past are looked at but produce no meaning. How this hurts! I strive to pry open a niche in her memory to bring some joy or laughter or some emotions but it is usually futile. She remains silent or blankly stares into my face I don't know what is going on but memory doesn't appear to be present. I retell the joys of our courtship so she can live again joy and happiness. I recall the 61 years of ministry around the world but there is no visible recognition of any of it.

They are engraved indelibly in my memory. Alzheimer's has burned them out of hers. What an insidious disease! Treasured moments are obliterated. Her eyes search my face. Her voice remains silent. Her emotions are unresponsive. She mumbles "I don't know". Tears blind my eyes. I am frustrated to the point of silence. I want to hear her laugh at our times of joy. I want to feel the warmth of her emotions. I need her arms around my neck bringing me comfort and strength for each day. They hang limply in her lap. I need to have her advice and to hear her pray for our ministry and me as of old. What to do?

Alzheimer's silently creeps in and pulls down the black curtain over memory. At first it is just a short black out. Doctors surmise the beginning of her Alzheimer's was the cause of the auto accident in May 2000. She remembers nothing about the accident or her injuries. Next Alzheimer's freezes the motor skills. So many times she has rested and inspired me with her piano and organ music. Soon her brain could not transmit to her hands to strike the right notes. It broke my heart when I had to suggest she be replaced playing for the assisted living facility worship services. I try to keep her singing but her eyes do not to focus quickly enough to send a message to formulate the words. Why does Alzheimer's have to take away everything?

Is she not entitled to some joys in the later stages of her life as she struggles with the inevitable? She no longer remembers how to function in the simplest household chores. She remembers nothing about how to cook the delicious meals, wash laundry, make a bed, or wash a dish. Participating in a stimulating event is no longer possible.

How am I to live my life and intrude into her darkened memory? I have no way of knowing what she understands, but I will maintain faith in my God. Psalm 136 says 26 times *"His love endures forever"*. That love opens the door to *"My grace is sufficient for you, for my power is made perfect in weakness. Therefore, I will boast all the more gladly about my weaknesses, so that Christ's power may rest upon me—for when I am weak, then I am strong"* (2 Corinthians 12:9,10). I will pray for and claim, *"to each one of us grace has been given as Christ apportioned it"* (Ephesians 4:7). I will tell and recall memorable events. I will make her laugh even though she may not understand everything. I will show her pictures and name the people in them. I will read to her and tell her about people both in the past and the present. I will encourage her friends to visit her. She may not communicate or understand everything but their presence stimulates her for the moment. I will take every opportunity to expose her to music. I will be delighted when I see happiness on her face and the music weaves its way into her mind. When she smiles at recognizing a tune or claps her hands in rhythm I am blessed.

Alzheimer's has reversed time. Erica is like a child who is yet to be exposed to experiences upon which memories are built. Paul write in I Corinthians 13: 11 *"When I was a child I talked like a child, I thought like a child, I reasoned as a child"*. but reminds us, *"I shall know fully, even as I am known"*. Until that time we will trust *"in the more excellent way"* which is *"Now these three things remain: faith, hope and love. But the greatest of these is love"* (I Corinthians 12:31 and 13:13).

Alzheimer's disease can blur the memory but once you love as we have loved the feelings continue to burn brightly. The love that made us one is unbroken even by Alzheimer's disease.

ALZHEIMER'S STEALS AGAIN

AUGUST 18, 2003

From the beginning God declared it was not good for man to be alone (Genesis 2:18). God created the wife to be beside the man. She was to be a companion ever by his side. She was to be his helpmate through all the experiences that were to come. They were to be one (Genesis 2:24).

When Erica and I were married 61 years ago we pledged to support and comfort each other *"in sickness and in health until death parted us"*. Through the years the companionship in times of illness was a big part of determination and courage to be healed. When Erica miscarried a baby on the mission filed, I held her hand and encouraged her. I assured her that it would come out all right. As the result of the miscarriage surgery was necessary. I was there, holding her hand, as she came out of the anesthesia. In the difficult childbirth of our sons, I was there to assure her of my love and support. We were one in the pain and the joy when our sons were born.

Through my seven surgical procedures she was there. Her face was the first to come into focus as I struggled to return to her. Through the agony of cancer and the effect of chemotherapy, her hand gave me courage to survive. It was her hand that stroked my aching head. She applied the cold clothes to my feverish brow. She spoke words of encouragement and her presence strengthened me. She squeezed my hand as pain flashed through my body. She was there! She was so vital to the healing process.

Now Alzheimer's has stolen her desire and ability to be there for me in the time of illness. Alzheimer's has blurred her sensitive spirit to my needs. This horrendous disease seems to have cut the cords of concern.

Recently I was quite ill requiring being in the hospital twice. I told her how ill I was. She looked at me. There seemed to be no registering of what I was saying. There were no words of concern. The hands did not move to grip mine. There was no reaching out to stroke my head. There were no reassuring words that things would be okay. For the first time she could not accompany me to the hospital. After a day I would return to occupy the same room in the Health Care Unit for four days. There was no mention of why I was there or question how I was feeling. Alzheimer's had ripped away from me another vital joy of being together. When I returned the second time from the hospital the apartment greeted me with silence. I was so alone! It is not her choice or mine that we are separated in the companionship of suffering. It is not her will not to speak. It is not her intention to not show her love by touch.

So what to do with another loss? The sensitivity cannot be restored. Erica cannot relearn the love and concern that had been a strong pillar of our life together. So what to do?

I am determined to reach out to her as she struggles in her world of numbness. She does not appear to have any pain. I presume that she is aware that things are not as we would want, although I have no way of knowing that. Erica must continue to hear my voice telling her of my love. My hand must continue to touch her head, her hair, her face and body so she will know that I am still there for her. I must derive my strength from the wonderful memories of when she was able to be my companion in suffering. These memories even now break open the fountain of tears as I rejoice in what I have had. Hatred for Alzheimer's rages in my being. I will not permit the fire of rage to quench my love for Erica.

I will find comfort and strength in the Father of compassion and the God of all comfort *"who comforts me in all troubles, so that I can comfort those in any trouble with the comfort I have received from God"* (2 Corinthian 1:3-5). I will rejoice in Isaiah 49:13-15 *"Shout for joy, o heavens; rejoice, O earth, burst into song, O mountains! For the Lord comforts his people and will have compassion on his afflicted ones. Though she may forget I will not forget you!"*

A friend in Arizona after describing the suffering of his wife sent these words—

> Although things are not perfect because of trial or pain
> Continue in thanksgiving; do not begin to blame.
> Even when the times are hard, fierce winds are bound to blow
> God is forever able. Hold on to what you know.
>
> Move out of "Camp Complaining". No weapon that is known
> On earth can yield the power praise can do alone.
> We'll run the race with gratitude, exalting God most high.
> Yes, there'll be times good and bad
> But, Zion waits in glory.
> Where none are ever sad!

HOUSECLEANING

SEPTEMBER 12, 2003

I am writing this on our 61st wedding anniversary. My emotions are bubbling up and hard to contain. As I bought her yellow roses the kind, motherly clerk wanted to know the occasion. I blubbered out the reason and Erica's disease. As I paid the clerk said, *"May I give you a hug to share with Erica?"* As I gave Erica the roses I asked if she remembered the significance of three roses. She stared at me with no apparent understanding. I reminded her *"the three mean I LOVE YOU"*. And I again assured her how very much. As I held her and kisses her I prayed, *"O, my Lord, will the pain ever cease?"*

In addition to the twice a month maid service the housecleaning service annually sends in a crew of ladies to deep clean the appliances, drapes and, rugs and to polish the furniture. This is such a blessing to us since Erica is no longer able to partner with me in doing these things.

In preparation for the annual cleaning I began to discard some items Erica no longer needed. As I opened drawers and shelves items popped out Erica had squirreled away for future use. Pain ripped me as I handled each item and discarded many. Some items were too painful and I gently laid them back to be handled another day. These items had been worthwhile to her. They were part of her treasure. Now Alzheimer's has spun the cobwebs of forgetfulness into her brain and she only can say *"I don't remember."* I know there are more painful days ahead.

I know that I must do some housecleaning of myself before I can be as helpful to Erica and cooperative with those who care for her. Paul wrote *"In a house there are articles; some are for noble (honorable) purposes and some for ignoble (dishonoring). If a man cleanses himself from the latter (ignoble), he will be an instrument for noble purposes, made holy, useful to the Master and prepared to do any good work"* (2 Timothy 2:20,21). Alzheimer's disease cuts and slashes the caregiver twenty-four hours a day. It is like a fire in tinder dry grass, sweeping over 36,000 per year into its fold and leaving the caregiver standing with only ashes and memories of what might have been.

Reflecting on myself I became aware that I was allowing the privilege of being a caregiver to corrode my spiritual life. I was becoming irritable with myself and those who give loving care to Erica. The dust of depression was settling down and clogging my understanding of the task of caring for my dear afflicted one. Irritability was weakening my ability to be what I must be. The trivial was being magnified and the worthwhile overlooked. I desire and expect the very best care for Erica possible. My ignoble attitudes will not change people who are only doing what is necessary.

My sensitivity to the difficult task of caring for those who no longer can make decisions, cannot speak coherently or care for themselves was becoming numb. It is time for some house cleaning of myself if I am to be *"a holy instrument for noble purposes, made holy, useful to the Master and prepared to do any good work"*. I was jolted back to be reminded that yellow roses are a sign of "joy". I must clean out that which is robbing me of the joy of the Lord and the joy of serving Erica and others.

An email asks the question "What is in your sponge?" When squeezed "what comes out?" Alzheimer's squeezes the caregiver! As it does, "What comes out?" Anger? Bitterness? Remorse? Irritability? Acceptance? Love? Jesus spoke to all when He said, *"clean the inside and then the outside also will be clean"* (Matthew 23:26). Paul calls upon us to *"purify ourselves from everything that contaminates the body and spirit, perfecting holiness and reverence for God" (2 Corinthians 7:1)*.

It is a nice feeling to have a clean house. It is a better felling to have a clean spirit and Christian attitude so I can fulfill Paul's words to Timothy (quoted above). I cannot change the ravages of Erica's disease. But I can, with God's help and the prayers support of God's people, make certain that my attitudes make it possible to *"be useful to the Master and prepared to do any good work"*.

If I fail to do this it will creep into my ability to love Erica and ways that show her that love. An 80 year old husband, whose wife had not known him for five years, continued to visit her, love her and be with her. He said *"True love is not physical, nor romantic. True love is acceptance of all that is, has been, will be, and will not be"*.

I love her more today that I did 61 years ago when she came down the aisle, clutching her bouquet of yellow roses, to be my beloved. She must know and feel that love today. Others need to know that I love her intensely and I want to minister to her and others out of love.

Today, I must pray *"cleanse me from secret faults "*(Psalm 19:12 K.J.V.). It must be my constant prayer *"Search me, O God, and know my heart; test me and know my anxious thoughts. See if there is any offensive way in me, and lead me in the way everlasting". (Psalm 139:23,24).*

ALONENESS

OCTOBER 15, 2003

I am sitting in a well-appointed hotel room 206 miles from Erica. Unfamiliar objects surround me waiting to be used. The only sound breaking the silence is the blaring TV in the next room. The smooth, unwrinkled, bed shrieks at me *"You are alone!"*.

I am with 140 senior adults who love Erica and me. Yet I am alone. I struggled for two months to get the consent of my mind and will to go on this trip without Erica. My peers encouraged me *"You need to go", "You need a break", "and It will do you good"*.

My mind responded, *"A break from what?* Alzheimer's has broken the connection. Yet, I need her! I need to be with her! I have no idea she comprehends what I am doing or what I am telling her. Sometimes she seems to understand briefly. I have never been on a trip like this without her. We have talked about what we were seeing and doing. All I see or do finds me saying to myself, *"Erica would love this. Erica would really enjoy this. Erica would be thrilled to see the flowers and sights"*.

Alzheimer's has confined her to a small bare room in an area of the Health Care Unit. I am alone! She is not able to be with me. She cannot enjoy this. Am I supposed to enjoy these things without her? For over 61 years being together made up our wonderful life. Friends surround me yet I want Erica to be beside me, to see what I am seeing, to enjoy the sights, sounds and food. I identify with the Psalmist *"I am like the desert owl, like an owl among the ruins. I lie awake. I have become like a bird alone on the roof"* (102:6,7).

Alzheimer's has made ruins of our wonderful life. Life has become a desert. I am like the bird perched on the roof looking down. I see couples laughing and talking as they go about. I see close friends chatting together. In the midst of a crowd I stand-alone. At meal times and events there is always a vacant chair beside me. I am alone. Erica is not there. An unwanted and uncontrollable disease has disconnected me from my most precious relationship.

God intended for man to be connected to someone to love and be loved in return. God created man and gave him plenty to occupy his time and energy. But God said, *"It is not good for man to be alone. I will make a helper suitable to him"* (Genesis 2:19). God declared this as being *"very good" (Genesis 1:31). The significance of bring connected is well stated in Ecclesiastes 4:9-12. "two are better than one".* The work is done better when two work together. They help each other when one falls. They keep each other warm. They defend and protect each other. Piece by piece Alzheimer's has rusted through the connection with Erica. I am alone.

The past has been blotted out of her mind. The present is clouded with uncertainty. The future is an impossibility. The disease is not reversible. It pushes the caregiver outside the normal connection and leaves me feeling alone.

Alzheimer's is not contagious. but some treat it as so. Some friends, once depended upon, have moved on to other matters which consume their time and efforts. The flood of encouraging letters, e-mails, and cards has become a trickle. The telephone, once ringing incessantly, now sits in silence. Social contacts are slow in coming. Visitors, once numerous, now are few. Inquiries about Erica are now only from the closest friends. I am alone. So where do I go now?

Jesus was often left alone in his trials and difficulties. Friends and family did not understand His struggles. Yet, he said to His closest friends, *"You will leave me all alone. Yet, I am not alone for the Father is with me"* (John 16:32). Then He promised, *"I tell you these things, so that in me you may have peace. In this world you will have trouble. But take heart! I have overcome* the world" (John 16:33). Earlier in the same conversation Jesus said, *"Now is your time of grief, but I will see you again and you will rejoice, and no one will take away your joy. Ask and you will receive, and your joy will be complete"* (John 16:22-24). He encourages me with these words *"Peace I leave with you; my peace I give you. I do not give to you as the world gives. Do not let your hearts be troubled and do not be afraid"* (John 14:27).

The pain of the disease gnaws at the caregiver. Aloneness is real to the caregiver. The pain is constant. I must look beyond the aloneness. I must believe that adversity cannot crush me if I look beyond myself to the Lord's assurances. I need to look for golden nuggets to be minded from the pit of aloneness. An unknown poet put it this way—

> "Looking back I clearly see
> All the grief that had to be
> Left me when the pain is o'er
> Richer than I'd been before."

Isaiah asked the question *"Can a mother forget the baby at her breast and have no compassion for the child she has born?"* The answer is "Yes". The Lord replies, *Though she may forget. I will not forget you" (Isaiah 49:15).* The Lord says the reason being *"I have made you, you are my servant, I will not forget you"* (Isaiah 44:21).. My prayer in the midst of my feeling of Aloneness becomes *"Do not cast me away when I am old, do not forsake me when my strength is gone"* (Psalm 71:9).

In my feeling of being alone. I take heart in these things –I have Jesus as my example. I have His promises to provide grace, strength and peace in my trials and times of aloneness.

I have the Father who promises, *"Never will I leave you; never will I forsake you, so I say with confidence, The Lord is my helper, I will not be afraid. What can man* (or Alzheimer's) *do to me?"* *(*Hebrews 13:5b, 6).

I have the Holy Spirit to reply upon to stand beside me as my Comforter and Helper and *"He will bring glory to me by taking what is mine and making it known to you"* (John 16:14).

I have the loving and praying friends who sustain me in prayer.

The feeling of being alone is defeated as I call upon the resources of God's promised and provided grace and strength.

TOGETHERNESS

OCTOBER 22, 2003

I feel frustrated! I pick up my pen. Words gush out. It has been a typical busy day. I began the day seeking daily grace and strength from the Lord for these troubled days. The supply never runs out. I do the laundry for Erica and me. I shop and fix two meals for myself. I take care of necessary business items. I assured myself the apartment was neat and clean as Erica kept it. I prepared for the three Bible studies I have this week. I exercised to keep my mind alert and body in tone. I did some writing on my books. I am tired!

I look at the clock. Unfinished tasks are laid aside. It is "togetherness" time. I have joyfully anticipated this all day. I go to be with Erica. I stay with her until the nursing aide puts her to bed. This is when I am ripped from her. This time of "togetherness" takes priority over everything. The unknown poet penned my feelings,

> "I love you, not only for what you are,
> But for what I am when I am with you
> I love you, not only for what
> You have made of yourself,
> But for what you are making of me".

When ministry calls me away I visit her before I leave and hurry back to be with her before she sleeps. I wrote in a new study Bible she wanted, *"To Erica—on being a reminder that you are my first priority in all of my life and a constant reminder of our life together and my love of each day"*.

When I arrive at the "togetherness" hour she flashes her beautiful smile at me. I kiss her! I hug her! I pat her! I tell her how much I love her. Sunshine breaks forth and brings joy into an ordinary tiring day. We are "together" again. The Hebrew word for "together" means, "become an unit". This is what God intended: *"For this reason a man will leave his father and mother and be united to his wife, and they will become one flesh"* (Genesis 2:24). The Greek word for "together" can be translated as "the same". This uniting— this sameness-- is God's design for a husband and wife. *"So they are no longer two, but one. Therefore what God has joined together, let man not separated"* (Matthew 19:6).

Paul voiced what should happen: *"My purpose is that they may be encouraged in heart and united in love, so that they have the full riches of complete understanding, in order that they may know the mystery of God, namely, Christ"* (Colossians 2:2).

What man is forbidden to do, Alzheimer's disease has done, Our 7 day, 24 hours a day, has been crushed into about 4 hours a day. In these precious hours I tell her what I have been doing. I read to her. I pray with her. I take her for rides in the car and we may stop for a Chinese or shrimp meal. I push her in the wheelchair outside in the sunshine and around the campus. I show her the flowers, animals and birds. We watch TV together. I take her to musical programs. At times we sit quietly holding hands. We are "together".

The time we are separated is not our choice The aide enters the room to say, "Mr. Morris, you want to leave now so I can put the two ladies to bed?" I tell Erica I must leave. She looks at me and asks, *"Do you want to go?"* I reply *"No!"* But I have no choice. I kiss her good night and tell her how much I love her. With tears in my eyes I hurry away and stumble to the lonely apartment. Togetherness is over for the day. I start anticipating tomorrow.

As I write these words I feel God's ministry of grace and peace flow gently into my stressed soul. The ring of the telephone startles me back to reality. It is my dear Chinese friend from Malaysia. He and his wife helped Erica and me begin the Baptist church in Sabah. *"Pastor Morris, we* have *not heard from you for sometimes. Are you all right? How is Erica? I want you to know how much the people in Malaysia appreciate the hard work you and Erica did to bring the Gospel to that area. We love you and*

Erica and pray daily for you. What can we do to help you? Please let us know".

As the call ended I saw a card just received from a busy young couple *who wrote to say "We just wanted to tell you that we love you and Erica and think and pray for you".* I felt warm and encouragement crowded out the depressed feeling...My "togetherness" with Erica is limited by factors I can't control. The arms of friends such as these help me continue to walk a rough path with a sense of abiding peace and strength for each day.

As I continue to reflect on "togetherness" memories boost my spirits. Our ministry together for over 61 years causes me to identify with Psalm 55:4::*"We took counsel together and walked into the house of the Lord"* (KJV). Erica and I have done just that in over twenty churches in five countries. Hundreds of times we have *"burst into song together"* (Isaiah 52:9). How I praise the Lord for the harmony in our spirits. When we are together there is a distinct feeling that we are not alone. *"For where two come together in my name, there am I with them",* said Jesus in Matthew 18:20.

As long as the Lord allows I will concur with William Shakespeare (Sonnet 116) entitled TRUE LOVE.
> "Let me not to the marriage of true minds
> Admit impediments. Love is not love
> Which alters when it alteration finds,
> Or bends with the remover to remove.
> O, no! it is an ever-fixed mark,
> That looks on tempest and is never shaken;
> It is the star to every wandering bark,
> Whose worth's unknown, although his height be taken.
> Love's not Time's fool, though rosy lips and cheeks
> Within his bending sickle's compass come;
> Love alters not with the brief hours and weeks,
> But bears it out even to the edge of doom.
> If this be error and upon me proved,
> I never writ, nor no man every loved."

THANKSLIVING

NOVEMBER 27, 2003

Coping with the uncertainties of Alzheimer's disease is an unending endurance test. Changes take place daily—even hourly. Inwardly I squeal with joy when Erica is alert, responsive, laughing and animated. I struggle with the desire to take her in my arms and bring her to our home. Like the ebb and flow of the tide she changes. I cry "Stop"! But the undertow tugs at me. I ache from the non-stop struggle. Daily I scramble for a firm footing for the moment. At times, I feel I will drown. I wasn't born to be a caregiver. I am a husband deeply in love with my wife, Erica. An email said, *"True love is neither physical, nor romantic. True love is an acceptance of all that is, has been, will be, and will not be"*.

Alzheimer's disease is described like grains of sand slowly trickling through the hand. It is impossible to stop the trickle. But I have the power to squeeze tightly the grains and get the very best out of what is left. I am determined to get the best for her and for myself as the sands of time trickle on.

Rosalind Carter, former first lady, said, *"There are only four kinds of people in the world—*

Those who have been a caregiver

Those who are currently a caregiver

Those who will be a caregiver

Those who will need a caregiver".

I don't want to be a caregiver. But I am! I didn't choose to be a caregiver. But I am! What can I do to extract the most good from a bad situation?

Today is Thanksgiving Day. What should I be thankful for this day? The word "thank" comes from the Greek word for grace (charis). It is an attitude! Gladys Bailey, a 100-year-old badly crippled lady said her secret of long life was. "Let my attitude be gratitude". It is acceptable (charis) to be thankful when enduring suffering (1 Peter 2:19,20). Paul reminds me. *"Be joyful always; pray continually, give thanks in all circumstances for this is God's will for us in Christ Jesus"* (1 Thessalonians 5:18).

David, in his psalm of thanks. called on God's people to-
> *"Give thanks to the Lord,*
> *Call upon his name;*
> *Make known his deeds,*
> *Sing praise to him."*

This should be done as we, *"Look to the Lord and his strength; seek his face always. Remember the wonders that he has done" (1 Chronicles 16:8-12).* Being thankful for what we have extracts the good from the bad.

Camila Henson Flinterman wrote *"the memories of days past and hope for tomorrow; the love that sustains us both, we are, most of all, thankful"* James 4:6 reminds me that God gives greater grace (thankfulness) as I allow the Holy Spirit to produce gratitude in the midst of the quagmire of the disease.

In the midst of being thankful I am determined to have an attitude of patience toward Erica. I will not be a partner to hasten her inability to function. I will not make her more of an invalid than she is. I thrill with every little sign of her ability to function, comprehend and respond. My heart leaps with joy with her effort to string words together. I am greatly encouraged as she reads aloud to me the words written on the cards she receives. It may be stumbling, like a child, but she reads. What music to my ears! Like a parent with a child I find joy in her taking a spoon or fork and moving it to her mouth as she eats. It may be wobbly but she finds her mouth. What an accomplishment! I make jokes and say funny things. Like the tinkle of a bell in the wind she laughs. I am so thrilled her mind is still functioning in a limited way. She follows intently as I point out and read the Scripture to her. Often she says, "That is nice". She is unable to buckle enough words together to pray aloud. She listens intently as I pray. She says "Amen" at the close. I watch her beat out the rhythm of the songs

I play on the car radio or those played in worship services. She cannot sing but she hears and feels the music. What a blessing!

According to science this will change. But for now she is still with me. Our love is intact. I tell her several times a day. I hug her for myself and for her friends. Often she will pat my hand and say, "I love you, too". What more can I expect at this stage? I am thankful for all she has been, what she is now and what I still have. I will continue to squeeze every drop of happiness from the sands of time. When change is required my Lord will give me grace to adjust again. For that I am thankful.

A DIFFERENT CHRISTMAS

DECEMBER 23, 2003

This is the first Christmas in 62 years Erica and I have been separated in the Christmas season. Memories of Christmas in Michigan, Illinois, Virginia and Washington, D.C. are recorded in photos and engraved in my memory. The joy of celebrating "first" Christmas with new believers in Malaysia, Singapore, the Philippine Islands and the island of Borneo has enriched our lives. The accents of Chinese, Indians and tribal people singing the carols either in broken English or their mother tongue, have made the true meaning of Christmas come alive. Carol singing, church worship services, candlelight communion, cheerful greetings, festive foods and exchanging gifts have made Christmas "merry".

Erica perfumed the home with the smell of goodies she made to give away. The furtive seeking for the right card and present to place at my breakfast place on Christmas day delighted her no end. Joy was very real in our home and world.

About four years ago an uninvited and most unexpected shadow began to enter our home. Alzheimer's disease with its sack full of troubles and problems arrived. The disease did not discriminate between who was "naughty or nice", as it began to empty its bag of disturbing symptoms. There is no way to recall or exchange the unwanted "gift".

Gone is the joy of hearing Erica play and sing the carols because signals are interrupted between eyes, brain, voice and fingers. No longer can she remember the recipes or how to mix the ingredients for the goodies. The thrill of reading and re-reading the beautiful cards and letters is now met with a blank stare and silence. Cuddling together, expressing joy and thanksgiving for the privilege of being together is met with no response. This is devastating to me! Her inability to put words together prevents her from say-

91

ing "thank you" as friends bring flowers, cookies and gifts. She has no feeling of joy or even looking at the presents. Her glazed eyes do not focus on my face. She no longer says, "I love you, too" in response to my expression of love. Day and night tears come. So how can this be a merry Christmas to me?

In reading again the stories of the first Christmas I am encouraged to discover that my struggle with this hateful disease is not unlike the conflicts that took place when Jesus was born. While the angels made heaven ring with *"good news of great joy" (Luke 2:10,14).* Mary was restless as she *"pondered in her heart"* (Luke 2:19) what this meant and the future for her child. Mary marveled at the words of Simeon praising God. But how many times did Mary worry about the unknown time when, *"A sword will pierce your own soul too"* (Luke 2:35)? The Magi from the east joyously presented gifts as an act of worship under the shadow of the impending slaughter of the innocent (Matthew 2:18). Apprehension and fear of the future was experienced by Mary (Luke 1:29) and Joseph (Matthew 1:20). Fear had to be crushed. Faith had to burst through as they came to experience Christ becoming *"Immanuel—God with us"* (Matthew 1:23).

Is this not a picture of how this dreadful disease cripples the patient and disrupts the family? Only the now is known. The future is fraught with apprehension and fear. Every word of the doctor is like the thrust of the coming sword. Every kindness of a caring staff is overshadowed by the dark future.

I fill waking hours with memories of Christmases past. My dreams are troubled by the shadowy figure of hopelessness for the future. My prayers batter the gate of heaven begging to become more like Jesus. I am committed to what I don't understand. I wrap myself in the cloak of His presence. The bright ribbon of daily hope ties Erica and me together, even as this despicable disease snips us apart. The stars twinkle brightly in the dark night of despair assuring me that the Lord, family and friends love us and there is light and hope. I am among those who are walking in darkness who *"have seen a great light; as those living in the land of the shadow of death, a light has dawned"* (Isaiah 9:2).

I pray for increased faith to follow to star to where Jesus is waiting to lift my burden. In my wavering moments I pray for the assurance to sweep over Erica and me so we will rejoice in Immanuel, who promises, *"Never will I leave you; never will I forsake you"* so we say with confidence, *"The Lord is my helper; I will not be afraid. What can man* (or disease) *do to me?"* (Hebrews 13:5b, 6).

His presence assures me that Christmases past are just that—past. Christmas present is wrapped in the joy of love for Erica and tied with the unbreakable ribbon, *"Peace, I leave with you, my peace I give to you. I do not give to you as the world gives. So let not your hearts be troubled and do not be afraid"*(John 14:27). I must live the Christmas present in *"My joy may be in you and that your joy may be completed and no one will take away your joy. Ask and you will receive and your joy will be complete"*. (John 15:11; 16:23,24).

Joy and Peace are the needed pieces in the jigsaw puzzle of living with this daily struggle. Only as I fit them into place will a beautiful understanding emerge. Erica is His and I am privileged to be beside her. Erica has brought so much light into my life for the past 62 years and I rejoice in that. Now I claim the promise which was given to the shepherds, *"Unto you in born a Savior. He is Christ the Lord"* (Luke 2:11). I need Him to daily save me from the crushing onslaught of this hated disease. And He will!!

A TRIBUTE

FEBRUARY 9, 2004

The head nurse of the Health Care Clinic, in passing, said, "Your wife has such elegant grace". "Wait a minute", I inquired, "What do you mean"? She stopped and said, "We minister to many patients with Alzheimer's disease. Erica has such elegant grace in her handling the disease. She is so easy to care for. She never complains. She never demands anything. She always smiles at us when we speak to her. She cooperates when we need her to do something. She has a radiant calmness about her. Her gracefulness and loveliness personifies the graces that God has provided her with and she has lived all her Christian life. She radiates a blend of all of God's graces. She gives meaning to the gifts of the Holy Spirit as told in Galatians 5:22,23, *The fruit of the Spirit is love, joy, peace, patience, kindness, goodness, faithfulness, gentleness and self control"*.

This tribute came after caring for Erica for nearly a year as a permanent resident in the Health Care Unit. It was no surprise to me that others had seen in Erica what I had been blessed with for nearly 62 years. I was, however, extremely grateful that others had seen what Erica would most desire to show to the world of suffering people.

I returned to the apartment with these comments buzzing in my mind. What is grace? Greek scholars reveal there are as many as 170 different words used in secular and religious Greek for the word: "grace". Each word is like a facet of a beautiful diamond ring each flashing a different hue of color. As all of the facets blend there is exquisite beauty. No single English word completely gives the full meaning to "grace".

The word seems to denote "external appearance". It speaks of the beauty or gracefulness of a person in charm of speech and thank-

94

fulness for blessings relating to God. It is a gift from God. Being in favor with God allows God's Spirit to dwell within us and produce characteristics of God. It is used as a synonym for the Spirit and interchangeably with "gifts of grace" and "gifts of the Spirit". James 4:6 promises God will give "greater grace" to the humble who turn away from the world.

Paul reminds us *"For it is by grace you have been saved, through faith-- and this not from yourselves, it is the gift of God—not by works, so that no one can boast. For we are God's workmanship, created in Christ Jesus to do good works, which God prepared in advance for us to do"* (Ephesians 2:8-10). The issue is not salvation but what I allow God to do in and through me. How far in advance? The word "advance" means "to cut forward a way". When God saved us he provided "sufficient grace" for each experience of life. He promised *"My grace is sufficient for you, for my power is made perfect in weakness"* (2 Corinthians 12:9).

God has deposited more than enough "grace" into each person's account. God sees and acts so as to meet the needs of the moment. When the dreaded disease of Alzheimer's thrusts itself into the mind, grace is ready. Erica's deposit is being unconsciously drawn upon as she wanders through the disease. She is receiving and showing *"But to each one of us grace has been given as Christ apportioned it" (Ephesians 4:7).* This is God's gift to her. She is *"attaining to the whole measure of the fullness of Christ" (Ephesians 4:13).*

The gift of grace is a manifestation of the Spirit *"given for the common good" (1 Corinthians 12:7). Tears* of joy fill my eyes because others are seeing this elegant grace in Erica.

She always has been and still is a beautiful person externally and most of all internally. She personifies the statement, "As the candle in a holy place, so is the beauty of an aged face". She is a literal manifestation of the grace of God in the life of a believer. She does not pretend to be—she is! This makes it possible for her to have elegant grace even in the grip of this most terrible disease.

I am convicted by the words of the nurse. How am I reacting to being the caregiver of such a beautiful person? Is the grace of God working in my daily attitudes and responses to the nurses, doctors and aids who attend to my lovely wife? Do I demonstrate that I am drawing from my deposit of grace? My prayer is, "O Lord, may the elegant grace seen in Erica radiate into my being! May I reflect God's grace toward her as she flounders under the influence of this disease?"

SPRING BRINGS GRIEF

MARCH 26, 2004

With a rush of tepid air spring announced its arrival. Brown twigs on the trees begin to twitch. The crocuses yawned their multi-colored arms out of hibernation. The narcissus and the jonquil raised their white and yellow trumpets and announced, "We're back! It is spring!" The white, purple and rosy hyacinths perfumed the air with their delicate aroma. The forsythia shook their bell shaped flowers and waved their long arms at every passerby. The pear trees lined the streets with their skirts of pure white. The ornamental cherry and peach trees splashed their delicate pink everywhere. The violets turned their multi-colored faces up and smiled to all. The snowball trees vied for attention with their fluffy white cotton like balls.

The robins hop-scotched across the lawn stopping every so often to cock their heads and listen for breakfast. They plunged their saber like beaks into the warming ground and pulled up their squirming morsels.

You can almost hear the buds as they pop open and display their leaves in various shades of green. All the color and beauty is painted against a sparkling blue sky. The sun reached down and kissed the dew coated electric wires and they shimmered into diamond necklaces draped between the stark wooden poles.

Spring is here! How joyous is the season with which God has graced us. It has always been Erica's favorite season. She longed for this glorious time when we were in the tropics. I am so excited! I hurry to bundle her into a wind-breaker and into the car. I want her to see, to feel, to smell this time of rebirth. I am eager for her to feel the warmth of the sun. I want her to bathe in the beauty around us. I want her to become intoxicated with the smell of the flowers. I tremble with the exciting thought of sharing with her this resurrection of God's creation.

But — Alzheimer's disease has clouded her brain. Spring cannot penetrate the jangled and twisted nerves of her brain. Her eyes see but do not see. She slumps in the car seat. I plead, "Honey, look at the flowers and the trees. Let all your senses drink deeply of what God is doing to the earth for us". There is no response! Her eyes are either closed or unseeing. Her emotions are deadened. Tears blur my eyes as I drive up and down the streets begging God to let her see, feel and enjoy spring. My heart aches to let her experience a child like delight in the moment. O, Lord, what can I do to bring back spring time to my dearest Erica.

The sun is shining but the dark clouds that have rolled in on Erica begin to smother me. The chilling frost is nibbling at my heart. The only music I hear is the monotonous dirge of the insidious disease. What can I do?

Lord, I cannot survive with this attitude. How helpless I feel. A lady with the dreaded disease in the health care looked at me with pleading eyes, "You are a minister. Can you not heal me of this?" I cannot bring spring into the mind that is snowed in with results of Alzheimer's disease. I cannot untwist the strands that strangle the ability to feel, see and respond. I am faced with a choice for myself and for my darling. God, give me the answer!

Proverbs 10:9 challenged me, *"The man of integrity walks securely, but he who takes crooked paths will be found out"* The Hebrews word for "integrity" means "completeness". The Psalmist translates the word as "blameless". *"I have trusted in the Lord without wavering—But I lead a blameless life; redeem me and be merciful to me, My feet stand on level ground; in the great assembly I will praise the Lord"* (26:1,11,12).

When Satan unleashed his worst against Job God said, *"He still maintains his integrity, though you incited me against him to ruin him without any reason" (Job 2:3).* Erica did nothing to deserve this insidious disease. Science cannot indicate a reason why it strikes some and not others. We only know it is here. The test, at this point, is on me.

Will I maintain integrity as the lashes of this disease scourge the mind of Erica and rip at my emotions? Job, suffering in the midst of his troubles, would say, *"Till I die, I will not deny my integrity. I will maintain my righteousness and never let it go; my conscience will not reproach me as long as I live" (27:5,6).* What confidence Job had in His God! He believed that God would bring good out of the dark clouds of trouble, if he maintained his integrity. He would live to see this fulfilled. *"The Lord blessed the later part of Job's life more than the first" (Job 41:11.*

Job suffered much. I am still suffering. Job lost much. I am still losing each day. Job did not blame God. Job did not accuse the environment, diet or inheritance. Job accepted the condition as his assignment for the hour. It has happened! Job believed God would bring blessings out of his troubles. He stood up against his wife. *"Shall we accept good from God, and not trouble? In all this, Job did not sin in what he said" (Job 2:10).* Job declared his friends as being *"as undependable as intermittent streams, as the streams that overflow when darkened by thawing ice and swollen with melting snow, but that cease to flow in the dry season, and in the heat vanish from their channels"* (Job 6:15-17).

It is my turn to prove my integrity. I rely upon God's grace to believe that God is still in control. I pray for strength to endure what I cannot change. I pray, like Job, *"Oh, that I might have my request, that God would grant what I hope for" (Job 6:8).*

I cannot bring back the springtime to Erica. It is not possible to refocus her eyes to see all that I see. This being so, I would pray for strength to say, as Job did, *"I would still have this consolation—my joy in everlasting pain—that I have not denied the words of the Holy One"* (Job 6:10).

LESSONS I AM LEARNING

FEBRUARY 12, 2004

For more than 4 years I have been a resentful student in the school for caregivers. There is no graduation because the course is never finished. What am I learning? Is the learning process equipping me to be a better caregiver to my beloved Erica? Have the journal entries been engraved on my heart and not just lines on paper? What am I learning about the disease and how to adjust to the persons who have been afflicted?

As a caregiver and volunteer chaplain in the Health Care Units I am learning that the persons suffering the ravages of Alzheimer's disease are still dignified, worthwhile and wonderful persons. They still have dignity and deserve respect from everyone. They may be like the denominational leader who recently said, "I have outlived myself". Yet, each day, he dresses in a gleaming white shirt, tie and suit as if he were going to a board meeting. He still has a good self-image. I must encourage that. An Alzheimer's patient is not just a lump of flesh confined to a wheel chair or room waiting for the funeral gurney to whisk their body away. Who they were in the past and who they are now must be protected and projected. Every day I want Erica dressed in her best clothes, I see that her hair is professionally cared for so she looks smart. She receives a weekly manicure from the aides. I insist she receive the best of care. She is still my wonderful soul mate and I want her respected and cared for.

I am instructed in how rapidly the disease is multiplying. 1 in 10 Americans have a family member afflicted. Nearly 5 million have the disease. The number is increasing rapidly. One-half of all patients in nursing homes have some form of Alzheimer's. It is the fourth largest cause of death in America. 10% of persons over 65, 20% of those over 75 and nearly 50% of those over 85 have the disease. I am to inform others of this scourge.

I am being informed of the large sum of money annually being spent to find a treatment for the disease. When the treatment is found it will delay the onset of the disease for at least 5 years and reduce the number 50% after 50 years. There are presently four drugs that may be helpful. It is necessary that I, as a caregiver, be alert to every possible medical assistance. I need to spread the word so others may be helped. The local chapter of the Alzheimer's Association is the best source of information and help.

One lesson I am learning every day is that grief is daily. There are days when I try to deny what is happening. Anger and guilt continue to flare up. Unexpected happenings plunge me into sadness and depression. The frustration of having no resolution leaves me squirming in my emotions. Moments of questioning the fairness of the disease cause me to churn inwardly. There is no closure in sight so there is no end to the grief process.

I am rejoicing in the complete sufficiency of God's Word, His all-sufficient grace and the peace prayer brings. This is the only source of survival. In each of my journal entries God has revealed just the right word to bring me back from despair and provide hope for Erica and me.

History teaches me that things like this just don't happen. God is not surprised nor unaware that Erica has Alzheimer's and that I am a caregiver. What happens because of what happens is the important issue. It is exciting to see God's hand at work as I accept this as His assignment for me at this time. The struggle ceases as I put my choice under the authority of God's Word and exercise faith in Him who makes no mistakes. The unknown poet wrote--

"I know not what the day may bring--
Tomorrow waits unknown;
But this I know, the changeless Christ,
My Lord, is on the throne."

I am learning to not soar off on a guilt trip because I have entrusted Erica to the continuing care of others. I am not failing my marriage vows. I am not abandoning Erica. I am learning to love her enough to let her go. Jesus, when He no longer could care for his mother, entrusted her into the hands of a beloved friend (John 19:26,27). The friend, out of deep compassion, took Jesus' mother as his own.

One of the nurses said to me, "Money or employment is not the reason we work here. It is out of compassion for Erica and others that we minister here". Her statement reassured me that love for Erica and the others was not limited to me. My love for Erica rages now more than ever. Because of this I am able to entrust her to others who can give her the care that I am unable to give.

I am continually instructing myself how to be a caregiver. Authorities maintain, "To be a good caregiver you need to take care of the caregiver". This is the most demanding lesson. It means that I must do something at times I don't want to do. I must entrust Erica to others and take a mini-break. Guilt has to be pushed down. Determination to have a ministry apart from Erica must be manifested. Enjoyment apart from Erica must be sought in the company of others. Distance is not to be measured in miles or hours. Relaxation, refreshment and renewal must be sought. Exercise of the body must be disciplined to keep the mind and emotions active. Ability to laugh at jokes and self must be practiced. I am learning to open myself up and let close friends catch a gleam of how I am hurting. I am learning to accept what I cannot change. I am praying for:

> Serenity to accept the things I cannot change
> Courage to change the things I can, and
> Wisdom to know the difference.

I am learning what Barbara de Angelia meant in her poem--

REAL MOMENTS

"Yesterday is history

Tomorrow is a mystery

Today is a gift

That's why we call it

THE PRESENT".

Erica's unwanted condition makes her a "now" person. The present moment is all she has. I am moving into that mode. Quality of time and togetherness is the most important.

I am experiencing the reality that there are a few friends that are my support system. I call them when I am hurting and need to talk. I arrange to be with them to talk and explain my feelings of frustration and grief. I impose on them when I need something done for Erica or me. They are those who "stick closer than a brother" (Proverbs 18:24). They are not many. They may not be family. In the Malay language there are several words for "friend". One word means "companion" and another "brother". The word "kawan" means one who is like a bee in a hive. They move together. The seek food together. They protect and fight for each other. They are together to the end. I have found those few. Some are near by and some are far away but they are always there for me. They are my support. I don't feel alone in my journey. I see it in their eyes as they visit and minister to Erica and me. I feel it in the small gestures they extend. I feel it in the grip of the hand or the hug from a young person, a male or female friend. I sense it in their demeanor toward me. I read it in the email, a specially chosen greeting card, or the unexpected telephone call from near by or 12,000 miles away. I am most fortunate to have these few "friends". Words are inadequate to express what they mean to me. They are jewels that glisten in the dark. They are gold nuggets that grace my soul.

I am still in the school. I am still learning. God is not finished with Erica or me.

THE VISIT

FEBRUARY 23, 2004

The parable of Jesus found in Matthew 25:34-46 instructs the disciples in ways believers are to minister as evidence of their love for Him. One-third of these ministries were *"you visited me"*. The Greek word translated "visit" means primarily "to inspect, to look upon or care for." In verse 43 he chastised those who *"did not look after me"*. Jesus equated visiting the needy and hurting as *"whatever you did for one of the least of these brothers of mine, you did for me" (verse 40),* and in verse 45 he said *"I tell you the truth, whatever you did not do for one of the least of these, you did not do for me"*.

Those who are unable to carry on normal activities are referred to as "shut in". By observation and research I find that Alzheimer's disease slams the door. and the patient, and often the caregiver or family, are "shut out". The afflicted may be o.k. physically. They may look fine. However, once the disease begins corroding the brain cells the afflicted become "shut out".

The unfortunate person is shut out from his/her normal self. The disease shuts out that person from memories. It disconnects the ability to function and enter into normal activities. Joyous occasions and normal relationships are limited. As one man sadly said, "I have outlived myself".

The disease shuts out the person from the family. He is limited in the ability to respond emotionally. She is handicapped in being able to embrace and return love to others. Family history is blacked out. There is no memory of how to respond to events, holidays, anniversaries or times of joy. Many reach the stage of being unable to comprehend or communicate. Eventually the disease destroys the ability to recognize family members. Some family members have great difficulty with this phase. The family is unable to cope with this limitation. One lady refused to visit her husband. When asked "why?" she replied, "He is dead! Why should I visit the dead?" On special occasions some family members bring flowers, candy or gifts. Often the patient can't appreciate or enjoy these. What the afflicted need is the presence of a loving person. Mother Teresa said, "The greatest suffering is to feel alone, unwanted, unloved". As a chaplain I am often asked by the Alzheimer's patient, "Where is my husband, my wife, my son or daughter?"

The church often shuts out the Alzheimer's victim. One man, who had been very involved in his church, put it this way "I have been put aside". A woman, who had been active for years, said, "I have been forgotten". A man said, "Since I became caregiver for my wife, the church has turned its back on us. I don't want to think they mean to or intend it that way, but they just do". One church, when assigning deacons to care for families, eliminated all the persons or families where there was Alzheimer's. "My mother was very active in our church", said the concerned daughter, "I am the organist and choir director of the church. No one of the staff has visited my mother since she came here. She would love to have someone pray with her. Will you pray with her every so often?" Why do the church, pastors, leaders and many members ignore the Alzheimer's person? The disease has broken talents and gifts. Some respond something like this, "We are building the kingdom. The patient, caregiver and family are non-functional. They cannot contribute to our program. They offer no gifts or talents to the ministry of the church. We are so busy taking care of those who are active or will return to be active we have little time for the inactive". Seldom is a pastor seen in the Alzheimer's unit. Leaders and members are so involved in their own circle of activities there is little effort to visit the Alzheimer's patient. A retired Episcopal Chaplain, of a continuing care home, said sadly, "People are dying for lack of attention and love in these homes".

Lisa P. Gwyther in her book,"*You Are One of Us*", *quotes* from the Alzheimer's Association of South Australia (1995) these three kinds of visitors—

> The *talkative* one who talks at the patient about persons the patient has long forgotten. The patient becomes confused and tired.
>
> Those who talk among *themselves*. They may include the caregiver but mostly they visit and ignore the patient. They often whisper to each other leaving the patient and caregiver wondering what is going on.
>
> The *visitors who plan ahead.* They plan ways to involve the patient. The conversation is directed to the patient. They are not disturbed by silence or long periods before a response is made. They make the patient smile or laugh. They express in words and manners affection to the patient. The patient is happy with the visit and relaxed.

Visiting is an art that everyone can learn. It should be practiced regularly and often. Some helpful suggestions *for visiting Alzheimer's patients are:*

DO

> ➤ Make an appointment and keep it, so patient and others are ready.
> ➤ Talk directly to the patient in a calm, regular voice.
> ➤ Be patient. It takes more time for the patient to respond.
> ➤ Be joyful. Praise the patient for how she looks or how he is doing.
> ➤ Be hopeful. The future is unknown.
> ➤ Express your love and affection. The patient still has feelings.
> ➤ Recall past achievements or activities of the patient.
> ➤ Introduce yourself to the patient.
> ➤ Have prayer with the patient, caregiver and family.

DON'T

- ❖ Ask the patient "Who am I?" or "Do you remember me."
- ❖ Ask questions of the patient. They may not know how to answer.
- ❖ Ask the patient to make choices or decisions.
- ❖ Stare at the clock, watch or appear to be bored.
- ❖ Talk about the patient as if she/he were not present.
- ❖ Belittle their condition or the care they are receiving.
- ❖ Talk baby talk or talk down to the patient.
- ❖ Talk about your problems. They have enough themselves.
- ❖ Argue with the patient
- ❖ Express pity for the patient, caregiver or family.

In the time Erica has been afflicted and I have been serving as chaplain the reasons people give for not visiting are disturbing. Some of the reasons that are given are:

Some think that Alzheimer's disease may be contagious and they don't wish to be exposed. It isn't!

Some feel that the disease someday may attack them and they don't like what they see.

Some do not handle suffering well so they don't want to be around suffering people.

Some who have had experiences with Alzheimer's, don't want the memories to be stirred up again.

Some do not know how to relate to a person who can't enter into a meaningful conversation.

Some cannot endure silence when the patient cannot speak.

Some are so busy with their own lives and living they have no time or interest in relating to one who can't enter their world.

Some do not believe the Alzheimer's patient can feel the presence of love or recognize them so it makes no difference whether they come or not.

Some feel that spending money on flowers, cards or gifts becomes too expensive in the length of time the Alzheimer's patient may live.

Some feel that since there is no hope of improvement they will just wait until the final visitation to show interest.

Some forget too soon who the patient was and what contribution they have made.

Some are so busy with church ministry to the active members they neglect those who are unable to improve.

Some forget that the patient is still physically present and needs love and compassion from caring people.

Some don't realize that the slightest attention is greatly appreciated by the patient, caregiver and family.

There isn't much we can do for the patient who has Alzheimer's disease, but what we can do we ought to do. Visiting is a small gesture showing great love for the patient, the caregiver and the family.

TALKING OR COMMUNICATING

MARCH 2, 2004

As Alzheimer's disease progresses the art of relating to the afflicted person becomes increasingly difficult. Each day can be a new challenge. Comprehension by the patient becomes weaker and weaker. When the connections in the brain are twisted and corroded it is a challenge to give and receive any meaningful reactions to speech each time I am with Erica.

Society and culture depend upon words and sounds for people to relate to each other. Spoken words do not always communicate.

The Greek word translated "talk" is "logos". It is "giving an account by word of mouth". It is never used in Greek for "to chat" or "chatter". The purpose of logos is "to give meaning". In John 1:1 the writer uses "logos". The context shows the Word as being Jesus who *"was with God and the Word was God. He was with God in the beginning"*. Jesus revealed God to us. When Phillip said, *"Lord, show us the Father and that will be enough for us"*, Jesus replied *"Anyone who has seen me has seen the Father—the words I say to you are not just my own"* (John 14:8-10).

Much talking today doesn't reveal any meaning. It fits into the description of Proverbs 16:23. *"Mere talk leads only to poverty"*. Kahlil Gibran said, "You can talk when you cease to be at peace with your thoughts".

Talking is the earliest sign we look for when our children are developing. The baby moves from unintelligible sounds to fashioning the word "mama" or "daddy". When this sound is made the parents jump with joy. The baby has expressed meaning to the relationship. Soon the child speaks sentences. Shortly the baby begins to communicate wants, like or dislikes and meaning. Desiderus Erasmus spoke of good talk as being, "When only such

110

things are spoken and heard as we can reflect upon afterwards with satisfaction; and without any mixture of shame or repentance". Much talk today does not measure up to these criteria.

Alzheimer's disease reverses the process. The patient's ability to form words regresses from sentences to a few disjointed words; to incomprehensible babbling; to gutturall sounds and crying and finally silence. What am I to do when these stages are reached?

I must find ways to communicate. The Greek word translated "communicate" means "to share in" or "to give a share to". Communication is "to share in or participate with". When talking is no longer possible, I must find ways to communicate with Erica. I need to remember that she does not need to be perfect to be loved. I must find ways to do what John Milton wrote:

"Apt words have power to suage
The tumors of a troubled mind".

"suage" suggests the specific ability to encourage easy and frictionless dealings with others.

The children of Israel struggling through difficult times depended upon God's promise and God's provision.

The promise was *"When you pass through the waters I will be with you, and through the rivers they shall not overwhelm you; when you walk through the fire you shall not be burned or scorched, nor shall the flame kindle upon you."*

The provision. *"Behold, I am doing a new thing. I will even make a way in the wilderness and rivers in the desert"* (Isaiah 43:2,19 The Amplified Bible).

As the Alzheimer's patient wanders in the wilderness of an uncontrollable disease, loving persons will find a way to provide rivers of communication in that desert experience.

111

Communication is more than talking and listening. It is a river on which I must sail into Erica's mind. It is an attitude that causes the desert to blossom In what ways do I communicate with Erica?

- The tone of my voice. calm, soft and normal.
- My facial expressions. Smiles convey feelings.
- Love words are always appropriate and understood.
- Touching. Gentle, light strokes on the hair or body.
- Rubbing the neck or back communicates love and affection. It relaxes her and she knows I care about her.
- Body language. Non-verbal gestures or pointing.
- Being relaxed makes her feel at ease.
- Efforts made to reach her. Look into her face and eyes. Point out flowers, cards, animals and birds.
- Spend time together. It may be silently holding hands.
- Listen to music together and commenting on what is heard.
- Comments on the weather, sunshine, rain, snow, flowers, or general topics without asking for a reply.
- Make her a part of what is going on in my life.
- Sharing pictures and talking about the past or present makes her feel a part of what I am doing.
- Sharing a piece of fruit together and talking about it.
- Share news about family and friends without expecting a reply.
- Recall and participate in spiritual things. Praying together, worshipping together, reading the Bible or some devotional thought together.
- Do things to make her smile and laugh together. Do funny things to make her laugh at me.
- Hold her in my arms when she is tense or nervous

I must remember that I do not know what she understands, what she is thinking or what she wants to communicate. I must be alert to watch carefully her non-verbal signs and try to interpret them. She will know we are communicating although words may not be spoken. I must not allow frustration to bubble up or become impatient with her.